···························
Cochlear and Brainstem Implants

....

Advances in
Oto-Rhino-Laryngology

Vol. 64

Series Editor

W. Arnold   Munich

KARGER

Cochlear and Brainstem Implants

Volume Editor

A.R. Møller   *Dallas, Tex.*

84 figures, 9 in color, and 4 tables, 2006

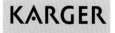

Basel · Freiburg · Paris · London · New York ·
Bangalore · Bangkok · Singapore · Tokyo · Sydney

. . . .

Aage R. Møller
School of Behavioral and Brain Sciences
University of Texas at Dallas, GR 41
PO Box 830688
Richardson, TX 75083-0688 (USA)

Library of Congress Cataloging-in-Publication Data

Cochlear and brainstem implants / volume editor, A. Møller.
    p. ; cm. – (Advances in oto-rhino-laryngology, ISSN 0065-3071
; v. 64)
  Includes bibliographical references and index.
  ISBN 3–8055–8157–2 (hard cover : alk. paper)
  1. Cochlear implants.   I. Møller, Aage R.   II. Series.
  [DNLM: 1. Auditory Brain Stem Implants.   2. Cochlear Implants.
  3. Auditory Brain Stem Implantation.   4. Cochlear Implantation.
  5. Hearing Loss–rehabilitation.   6. Hearing Loss–surgery.
  W1 AD701 v.64 2006 / WV 274 C6588 2006]
  RF305.C59 2006
  617.8′82–dc22

    2006014158

    Bibliographic Indices. This publication is listed in bibliographic services, including Current Contents® and Index Medicus.

© Copyright 2006 by S. Karger AG, P.O. Box, CH–4009 Basel (Switzerland)
www.karger.com
Printed in Switzerland on acid-free paper by Reinhardt Druck, Basel
ISSN 0065–3071
ISBN-10: 3–8055–8157–2
ISBN-13: 978–8055–8157–8

Contents

....

Introduction

Cochlear implants are now the most successful of all prostheses of the nervous system. Cochlear implants can provide good discrimination of speech and environmental sounds and some discrimination of music. Knowledge about the optimal time of implantation in children (sensitive periods) has improved the results of cochlear implants in children. Cochlear implants are used in individuals who are deaf or have severe hearing loss caused by loss of cochlear hair cells. Auditory brainstem implants (ABIs) provide stimulation of the cochlear nucleus and are used in individuals whose auditory nerves do not function. Until recently, ABIs were almost exclusively used in adults who had been operated on to remove bilateral vestibular schwannoma because of neurofibromatosis type 2. Used in such patients, ABIs have been less successful than cochlear implants in providing good speech discrimination. However, recently ABIs have been used in patients with other causes of auditory nerve dysfunction and in patients with deformed cochlea in whom it is not possible to perform cochlear implantation. In such individuals and in patients who have had their auditory nerve transected through head trauma and in children with congenital auditory nerve disorders (auditory nerve aplasia), ABIs provide similar speech discrimination as cochlear implants used in individuals with hearing loss of cochlear origin. This recent finding will undoubtedly widen the use of ABIs.

Cochlea implants activate the auditory nerve in the cochlea and thereby bypass sensory transduction in the inner hair cells, and more importantly, the complex function of the basilar membrane as a spectrum analyzer as well as that of the outer hair cells that provide automatic gain control. These functions were regarded to be fundamental for hearing. Frequency analysis performed by the basilar membrane was regarded to be the basis for auditory frequency discrimination that plays an important role in discrimination of sounds such as speech sounds.

When cochlear implants were first introduced, it was met with great disbelief that devices that bypassed the complex function of the cochlea could provide any useful hearing. While early cochlear implants using only one electrode did not provide speech discrimination in the way it is normally understood, the modern multielectrode implants can provide good speech discrimination, although multielectrode implants do not replicate the fine spectral analysis that normally occurs in the cochlea. It was even more surprising that good speech discrimination could be achieved with cochlear implants that only provide information about the spectrum of sounds without coding the temporal information in the sound waves, which has been regarded to be of fundamental importance for speech discrimination.

The book provides the clinical and scientific basis for cochlear and brainstem implants. The function, implementation and use of such prostheses are the topics of individual papers in the book.

The first paper by Roland and Wright discusses surgical aspects of cochlear implants. It describes techniques of inserting the electrode array using different entry points to the cochlea. This paper also discusses implantation in patients with residual hearing. Nadol and Eddington discuss histopatholgical aspects related to cochlear implants. Geers explains the influence of cochlear implants on language development in children and the effect of the age at implantation.

Although cochlear implants have been in practical use for many years, there are many aspects that need to be clarified. One such aspect is the importance of neural plasticity, which is discussed in detail in two papers. Sharma and Dorman discuss the development of the auditory system and the role of expression of neural plasticity in children with cochlear implants, and Kral and Tillein discuss the basic principles of neural plasticity applied to the auditory system and the principles of sensitive periods. These authors explain the critical periods in children for achieving optimal results. Loizou provides a detailed description of processors and the algorithms used in modern cochlear implants using the principle of the channel vocoder.

The next three papers are devoted to ABIs. Fayad and co-authors explain the surgical aspects of ABIs in patients with neurofibromatosis type 2, and Nevison describes methods for intraoperative testing of ABIs. Colletti discusses results of the use of ABIs in patients with other causes of auditory nerve injuries than bilateral vestibular schwannoma.

Two papers concern physiological aspects of cochlear and auditory brainstem implants. Shepherd and McCreery describe the basis for electrical stimulation of neural tissue and Møller discusses the neurophysiologic basis for cochlear and brainstem implants.

Acknowledgments

I thank S. Karger AG for making it possible to publish this book on the important topic of cochlear and brainstem implants. I want to thank Susanna Ludwig, Product Manager, and Elizabeth Anyawike, of the Production Team for their excellent work on this book. The Publisher and I also want to thank Advanced Bionics Corp. for the generous support that made it possible to reproduce some illustrations in color.

Aage R. Møller, Volume Editor
Dallas, May 2006

Møller AR (ed): Cochlear and Brainstem Implants.
Adv Otorhinolaryngol. Basel, Karger, 2006, vol 64, pp 1–10

....

History of Cochlear Implants and Auditory Brainstem Implants

Aage R. Møller

School of Behavioral and Brain Sciences, University of Texas at Dallas,
Dallas, Tex., USA

Abstract

Cochlear implants have evolved during the past 30 years from the single-electrode device introduced by Dr. William House, to the multi-electrode devices with complex digital signal processing that are in use now. This paper describes the history of the development of cochlear implants and auditory brainstem implants (ABIs). The designs of modern cochlear and auditory brainstem implants are described, and the different strategies of signal processing that are in use in these devices are discussed. The primary purpose of cochlear implants was to provide sound awareness in deaf individuals. Modern cochlear implants provide much more, including good speech comprehension, and even allow conversing on the telephone. ABIs that stimulate the cochlear nucleus were originally used only in patients with neurofibromatosis type 2 who had lost hearing due to removal of bilateral vestibular schwannoma. In such patients, ABIs provided sound awareness and some discrimination of speech. Recently, similar degrees of speech discrimination as achieved with cochlear implants have been obtained when ABIs were used in patients who had lost function of their auditory nerve on both sides for other reasons such as trauma and atresia of the internal auditory meatus.

Cochlear Implants

When Dr. William House [1] first introduced the cochlear implant it was met with great skepticism. Pioneering work by Michaelson regarding stimulation of the cochlea preceded the first clinical application of this technique [2]. While the success of modern multichannel cochlear implants is a result of technological developments, this success would not have been achieved, at least not as rapidly, if brave individuals such as Dr. House had not taken the bold step to try to provide some form of hearing sensations for individuals who were deaf because of injuries to cochlear hair cells.

Published studies of electrical stimulation of the auditory nerve date back half a century when Djourno and Eyries [3] described how electrical current passed through the auditory nerve in an individual with a deaf ear could cause sound sensation although only noise of cricket-like sounds. Later, Simmons et al. [4] showed that electrical stimulation of the intracranial portion of the auditory nerve using a bipolar stimulating electrode could produce a sensation of sound and some discrimination of the pitch of the stimulus impulses below 1,000 pulses per second (pps) with a difference limen of 5 pps. Above 1,000 pps, the discrimination of pitch was absent but the participant in the test could distinguish between rising and falling pulse rates.

The earliest cochlear implants used a single electrode placed inside the cochlea [1]. Introduction of cochlear implants that use multiple implanted electrodes and better processing of the signals from the microphone provided major improvements in speech discrimination. Using more than one electrode made it possible to stimulate different parts of the cochlea and thereby different populations of auditory nerve fibers with electrical signals derived from different frequency bands of sounds. Now, all contemporary cochlear implants separate the sound spectrum using bandpass filters so that the different electrodes are activated by different parts of the sound spectrum [5]. When such more sophisticated processing of sound was added the results were clearly astonishing, and modern cochlear implants can provide speech discrimination under normal environmental conditions [6]. Even those individuals who had great expectations were surprised by these accomplishments.

Sound Processing in Cochlear Implants

All modern cochlear implant devices process sounds and these processors have contributed greatly to the success of cochlear implants and auditory brainstem implants (ABIs). The advent of fast microprocessors, similar to what is found in personal computers, has made it possible to perform sophisticated signal processing of the sounds that are picked up by a microphone. Processors of modern cochlear and brainstem implants operate on the sounds picked up by the wearer's microphone. Refining the way the processors work and especially the algorithms used that has occurred during past one or two decades has contributed considerably to the success of cochlear implants. These processors have undergone many stages in their evolution since Dr. House introduced the first cochlear implants.

The processors of the first cochlear implants converted sound into a high-frequency signal that was applied to a single electrode in the cochlea. Contemporary cochlear implants have an array of several electrodes implanted

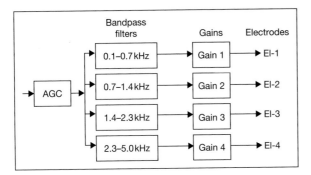

Fig. 1. Four-channel cochlear implant processor using the compressed analog princi-ples. The signal is first compressed using an AGC, and then filtered into four contiguous frequency bands, with center frequencies at 0.5, 1, 2, and 3.4 kHz. The filtered waveforms go through adjustable gain controls and are then sent directly through a percutaneous connec-tion to four intracochlear electrodes. Modified from Loizou [5].

in the cochlea so that the different electrodes stimulate auditory nerves along the basilar membrane, and processors that separate the sound spectrum using bandpass filters so that the different electrodes are activated by different parts of the sound spectrum. The dynamic range of electrical stimulation of auditory nerve fibers is much smaller than that of the normal activation through stimula-tion of cochlear hair cells; therefore, cochlear implant processors must com-press the range of sound intensities (automatic gain control, AGC) before it is applied to the bank of bandpass filters. Also the output of the bandpass filters is often subjected to some form of gain control.

In the simplest version of processors for multichannel cochlear implants, the spectrum of the signals from the microphone is divided into 4–8 frequency bands by a bank of bandpass filters. The output of these filters is applied to the respec-tive electrodes after AGC (fig. 1). This type of processors (known as the com-pressed analog, CA principle) presents both spectral and temporal information to the implanted electrodes and thus both spectral and temporal information become coded in the discharge pattern of the stimulated nerve fibers. (The CA approach was originally used in the Ineraid device manufactured by Symbion, Inc., Utah, USA [7]. The CA approach was also used in a UCSF/Storz device, which is now discontinued.)

Electrical interaction (cross-talk) between the electrodes that are implanted in the cochlea reduced the actual channel separation in the cochlear implants that used the CA principle. To solve this problem, short electrical impulses were applied to the different electrodes of the cochlear implants instead of (analog) signals from the bandpass filters and the different electrodes were activated

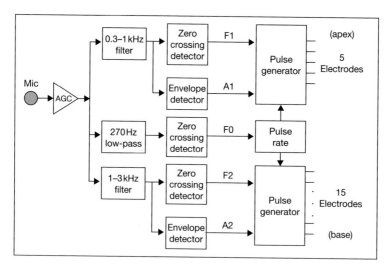

Fig. 2. Block diagram of the F0/F1/F2 processor. Two electrodes are used for pulsatile stimulation, one corresponding to the F1 frequency and the other corresponding to the frequency of F2. The rate of the impulses is that of F0 for voiced sounds, and a quasi-random rate (average of 100 pps) for unvoiced segments. From Loizou [5].

with small time intervals (continuous interleaved sampling, CIS) [5, 8; see also Loizou, this vol, pp 109–143]. The output of the bandpass filters controlled the amplitude of the impulses that were applied to the implanted electrodes. One manufacturer (Clarion) offers devices with processors that can be programmed with either the CA strategy or the CIS strategy. A modified CIS strategy, the enhanced CIS, is used in cochlear implants manufactured by the Philips Corporation under the name of LAURA [9].

With the progress in the sophistication of digital processing technology, the processors grew more and more complex and some of them analyze the sounds in detail and provide information about such features as formant frequencies of vowels and code that in the train of impulses that are applied to the implanted electrodes. The output of these processors was coded in electrical impulses that were applied to the electrodes in the implants. Introduction of these processors implied a fundamentally different approach from the CA or CIS principles of processing described above, although they used the CIS principle for applying the impulses to the stimulating electrodes. (Processors such as the Nucleus device that employ such feature extraction were introduced in the 1980s.)

Other processors especially designed for enhancing speech discrimination were developed for the Nucleus device in the early 1980s (fig. 2). These processors use a combination of temporal and spectral coding (known as the F0/F1/F2

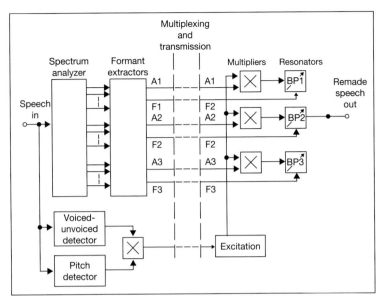

Fig. 3. Schematic diagram of a vocoder that was developed in the early 1960s. From Schroeder [10].

strategy). The fundamental (voice) frequency (F0) and the first and second formant (F1 and F2) were extracted from the speech signal using zero crossing detectors; F0 was extracted from the output of a 270-Hz low-pass filter, and F2 was extracted from the output of a 1,000- to 4,000-Hz bandpass filter (fig. 2). In a Nucleus device, the output of the processor controls the impulses that are applied to the implanted 22-electrode array. Another variant of this kind of processors, known as the MPEAK strategy, also extracts the fundamental frequency (F0) and the formant frequencies (F1 and F2) code the information in the pattern of the impulses that are applied to the implanted electrodes.

The algorithms used in these cochlear implant processors performed similar analysis as was developed half a century ago for use in analysis-synthesis telephony systems [10] (fig. 3). The goal was to provide continuous measures of features of speech sounds such as formant frequencies, the fundamental frequency of voiced sounds and information about fricative consonants, etc. to be sent to the receiver where it was used for synthesizing the speech. When used in cochlear implant processors, these complex systems did not live up to the expectations because they did work well in noisy environments [5], which often is present in connection with normal listening conditions. Background noise was not a concern for the development of telephony systems.

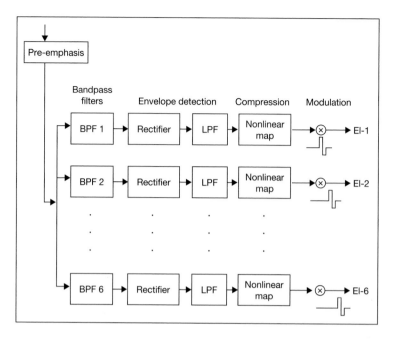

Fig. 4. Block diagram of a processor of the channel vocoder type that uses the CIS strategy in cochlear implants. The signal is first passed through a network that changes the spectrum (pre-emphasis) and then filtered in 6 bands. The envelope of the output of these six filters is full-wave rectified and low pass filtered. The low-pass filters are typically set at 200- or 400-Hz cut-off frequency. The amplitude of the envelope is compressed and then used to modulate the amplitude of biphasic impulses that are transmitted to the electrodes in an interleaved fashion. Modified from Loizou [5].

These kinds of processors were subsequently abandoned by most manufactures of cochlear implants because of the disappointing results in noisy environments and less complex systems were developed. These new strategies are based solely on information about the energy in a few frequency bands and the information about the temporal pattern is not used. Information about the energy in a few (6–10) frequency bands together with the smoothed temporal pattern of the envelope of the output of these bandpass filters is coded in the impulses that are applied to the implanted electrodes (fig. 4).

These systems that are known as channel vocoder-type processors, are now the most common type of processors in cochlear implant devices. The paper by Loizou [this vol, pp 109–143] provides a detailed description of processors that use the principles of the channel vocoder principle including variations of that strategy. One of these schemes, known as the Spectral Maxima Sound Processor treats all sounds equally and determines spectral maxima on the basis of the output of 16 bandpass filters. The output of the 6 bandpass filters with the largest amplitudes modulates the amplitude of biphasic impulses with a constant rate of 250 pps. These impulses are applied to the electrodes in the cochlea. A similar analysis scheme, the spectral peak strategy uses 20 filters instead of 16. For details about these processing strategies, see Loizou [5]. Many other strategies have emerged during recent years not only to improve speech discrimination but also to improve perception of other kinds of sounds, especially music. Some of these developments are discussed in the paper by Loizou [this vol].

Selection of Patients for Cochlear Implants

The success of cochlear implants depends on the selection criteria and these have changed over years. When cochlear implants first became available, only individuals who were essentially deaf (profound sensorineural hearing loss) received cochlear implants, and it took a long time before young children were given implants. More recently, a broader indication is accepted [11, 12] because it has become evident that individuals with severe hearing loss can benefit from cochlear implants. Bilateral implantation is now accepted. It is now regarded to be essential to provide cochlear implants to children as young as possible [13, 14; see also Sharma and Dorman, this vol, pp 66–88, and Kral and Tillein, this vol, pp 89–108].

Understanding the cause of hearing loss is important for selection of candidates for cochlear implants. Cochlear implants should naturally not be considered for individuals who have hearing loss caused by auditory nerve pathologies, for example individuals who have had bilateral vestibular schwannoma removed. Cochlear implants should not be given to children with auditory nerve aplasia caused by a narrow internal auditory canal, or trauma causing interruption of the auditory nerve [15]. Such children should instead have ABIs [Shepherd and McCreery, this vol, pp 186–205]. Candidates for cochlear implants should have appropriate examination and tests to exclude auditory nerve disorders as a cause of their deafness including an MRI scan that shows the structure of the internal auditory canal and not only the anatomy of the middle and inner ear [16]. ABIs should also be considered for individuals with hearing loss from injuries caused by trauma or diseases affecting the auditory nerve (auditory neuropathy) [Shepherd and McCreery, this vol, pp 186–205].

Auditory Brainstem Implants

Early studies of electrical stimulation of the inferior colliculus in humans did not provide any sensation of sound [4]. However, Colletti et al. [17] recently implanted electrodes in the inferior colliculus in a patient with bilateral auditory nerve section from bilateral vestibular schwannoma removal, demonstrating that electrical stimulation of the inferior colliculus can indeed provide sound sensation and some comprehension of speech.

William House and his colleagues at the House Ear Institute in Los Angeles [18, 19] introduced the use of a prosthesis that stimulated the cochlear nucleus electrically through an array of electrodes placed on the surface of the cochlear nucleus. These devices became known as ABIs. Before introduction of the ABI, it was shown that electrical stimulation of the cochlear nucleus in humans could produce auditory sensations [20].

Placement of the Electrode Array

ABIs use an array of approximately 20 electrodes placed on a plastic sheet. The electrode array is placed in the lateral recess of the fourth ventricle through the foramen of Luschka [21] in a similar way as electrodes that have been used for recording evoked potentials from the cochlear nucleus in neurosurgical operations [21–23]. Placement of an electrode array on the surface of the cochlear nucleus [Fayad et al., this vol, pp 144–153] is technically more demanding than placements of electrodes in the cochlea. Not only is it more difficult to maintain a stable electrode placement of electrodes in the brain than in the cochlea, but also it is also more difficult to place the electrode array so that an optimal population of nerve cells is stimulated. The use of electrophysiological methods for guiding positioning of electrode arrays is now widely used [15, 24; see also Nevison, this vol, pp 154–166].

Processors

Processors used in connection with ABIs use similar strategy as those used in cochlear implants. However, as more information about stimulation of the cochlear nucleus is obtained it may be expected that specialized strategies for processing of sounds for ABIs will be developed.

Selection of Candidates for ABIs

When first introduced, ABIs were almost exclusively used in patients with neurofibromatosis type 2 who had bilateral vestibular schwannoma removed. More recently, ABIs have been used in patients with bilateral traumatic injuries to the auditory nerve [15, 25, 26] and in children with malfunction of the auditory nerve such as may occur from internal auditory meatus malformation (atresia) causing auditory nerve aplasia [26]. ABIs are also now used in patients with cochlea malformation preventing implantation of electrodes [Shepherd and McCreery, this vol, pp 186–205]. While the results of ABIs in patients with bilateral tumors were disappointing, the results obtained in patients with other causes of auditory nerve injuries are similar to those obtained in patients with cochlear implants.

References

1   House WH: Cochlear implants. Ann Otol Rhinol Laryngol 1976;85(suppl 27):3–91.
2   Michaelson RP: Stimulation of the human cochlea. Arch Otolaryngol 1971;93:317–323.
3   Djourno A, Eyries C: Prothese auditive par excitatiob electrique a distance du nerf sensoriel a l'aide d'un bobinage inclus a demeure. Presse Med 1957;35:1417.
4   Simmons FB, Mongeon CJ, Lewis WR, Huntington DA: Electrical stimulation of acoustical nerve and inferior colliculus. Arch Otolaryngol 1964;79:559–567.
5   Loizou PC: Introduction to cochlear implants. IEEE Signal Processing Magazine 1998; 101–130.
6   Dorman MF, Loizou PC, Kemp LL, Kirk KI: Word recognition by children listening to speech processed into a small number of channels: data from normal-hearing children and children with cochlear implants. Ear Hear 2000;21:590–596.
7   Eddington D: Speech discrimination in deaf subjects with cochlear implants. J Acoust Soc Am 1980;68:885–891.
8   White M, Merzenich M, Gardi J: Multichannel cochlear implants: Channel interaction and processor design. Arch Otolaryngol 1984;110:493–501.
9   Peeters S, Offeciers FE, Kinsbergen J, Van Durme M, Van Enis P, Dykmans P, Bouchataoui I: A digital speech processor and various encoding strategies for cochlear implants. Prog Brain Res 1993;97:283–291.
10   Schroeder M: Vocoders: analysis and synthesis of speech. Proc IEEE 1966;54:720–734.
11   Quaranta N, Bartoli R, Quaranta A: Cochlear implants: indications in groups of patients with borderline indications. A review. Acta Otolaryngol Suppl 2004;552(suppl):68–73.
12   Cohen NL: Cochlear implant candidacy and surgical considerations. Audiol Neurootol 2004;9: 197–202.
13   Sharma A, Dorman MF, Kral A: The influence of a sensitive period on central auditory development in children with unilateral and bilateral cochlear implants. Hear Res 2005;203: 134–143.
14   Kral A, Hartmann R, Tillein J, Heid S, Klinke R: Delayed maturation and sensitive periods in the auditory cortex. Audiol Neurootol 2001;6.
15   Colletti V, Carner M, Miorelli V, Guida M, Colletti L, Fiorino F: Auditory brainstem implant (ABI): new frontiers in adults and children. Otolaryngol Head Neck Surg 2005.
16   Gray RF, Ray J, Baguley DM, Vanat Z, Begg J, Phelps PD: Cochlear implant failure due to unexpected absence of the eighth nerve – a cautionary tale. J Laryngol Otol 1998;112:646–649.
17   Colletti V, et al: Report on the first case of successful electrical stimulation of the inferior colliculus in a patient with NF2. In 5th Asia Pacific Symposium on Cochlear Implant and Related Sciences (APSCI 2005). Hong Kong, 2005.
18   Brackmann DE, Hitselberger WE, Nelson RA, Moore J, Waring MD, Portillo F, Shannon RV, Telischi FF: Auditory brainstem implant: 1. Issues in surgical implantation. Otolaryngol Head Neck Surg 1993;108:624–633.

19   Portillo F, Nelson RA, Brackmann DE, Hitselberger WE, Shannon RV, Waring MD, Moore JK: Auditory brain stem implant: electrical stimulation of the human cochlear nucleus. Adv Otorhinolaryngol 1993;48:248–252.

20   McElveen JTJ, Hitselberger WE, House WF, Mobley JP, Terr LI: Electrical stimulation of cochlear nucleus in man. Am J Otol 1985;(suppl):88–91.

21   Kuroki A, Møller AR: Microsurgical anatomy around the foramen of Luschka with reference to intraoperative recording of auditory evoked potentials from the cochlear nuclei. J Neurosurg 1995;933–939.

22   Møller AR: Intraoperative neurophysiologic monitoring. Luxembourg, Harwood Academic Publishers, 1995.

23   Møller AR, Jannetta PJ: Auditory evoked potentials recorded from the cochlear nucleus and its vicinity in man. J Neurosurg 1983;59:1013–1018.

24   Waring MD: Intraoperative electrophysiologic monitoring to assist placement of auditory brain stem implant. Ann Otorhinolaryngol 1995;166(suppl):33–36.

25   Colletti V, Fiorino FG, Sacchetto L, Miorelli V, Carner M: Hearing habilitation with auditory brainstem implantation in two children with cochlear nerve aplasia. Int J Pediatr Otorhinolaryngol 2001;60:99–111.

26   Colletti V, Carner M, Fiorino F, Sacchetto L, Morelli V, Orsi A, Cilurzo F, Pacini L: Hearing restoration with auditory brainstem implant in three children with cochlear nerve aplasia. Otol Neurotol 2002;23:682–693.

Aage R. Møller, PhD
School of Behavioral and Brain Sciences
University of Texas at Dallas, GR 41
PO Box 830688
Richardson, TX 75083-0688 (USA)
Tel. +1 972 883 2313, Fax +1 972 883 2310, E-Mail amoller@utdallas.edu

Møller AR (ed): Cochlear and Brainstem Implants.
Adv Otorhinolaryngol. Basel, Karger, 2006, vol 64, pp 11–30

. . . .

Surgical Aspects of Cochlear Implantation: Mechanisms of Insertional Trauma

Peter S. Roland[a], *Charles G. Wright*[a,b]

[a]Department of Otolaryngology, Head and Neck Surgery, University of Texas Southwestern Medical Center, [b]Callier Center for Communication Disorders, School of Behavioral and Brain Sciences, University of Texas at Dallas, Dallas, Tex., USA

Abstract

The development of hybrid electroacoustic devices has made conservation of residual hearing an important goal in cochlear implant surgery. Our laboratory has recently conducted anatomical studies directed toward better understanding mechanisms underlying loss of residual hearing associated with electrode insertion. This paper provides an overview of observations based on microdissection, scanning electron microscopy and temporal bone histology relating to inner ear injury that may occur during implant surgery. Trauma to cochlear structures including lateral wall tissues, the basilar membrane, the osseous spiral lamina and the modiolus is considered in relation to the implications of specific types of injury for hearing preservation. These findings are relevant to the design of future implant devices and to various important issues regarding the surgical technique used for implantation, including the possible use of the round window as a portal of entry for electrode insertion.

Copyright © 2006 S. Karger AG, Basel

Inner ear injury associated with insertion of electrode arrays has been a subject of concern since the inception of cochlear implant surgery. That concern rests on the supposition that the primary or secondary effects of insertional trauma may threaten the long-term survival of cochlear neurons, which must remain viable in order to be responsive to electrical stimulation [1]. There has recently been increased emphasis on the need to minimize insertional trauma so as to conserve hearing in implant recipients who retain significant levels of auditory function. This is especially true for patients who may be candidates for combined electrical and acoustic stimulation, in whom preservation of residual hearing is a primary goal [2].

Efforts are therefore underway to develop new electrode arrays having mechanical properties that permit optimal positioning of the array inside the cochlea and also reduce the occurrence of insertional injury. However, even with the best available devices and use of great care during surgical placement of electrode arrays, residual hearing is completely lost in at least 10–20% of patients receiving cochlear implants [3, 4]. The specific causes for the hearing loss in this group of patients are doubtless varied and they are not yet completely understood. However, direct mechanical injury of cochlear structures during electrode insertion seems likely to be a major factor.

Recent human temporal bone studies from our laboratory have focused on better understanding of mechanisms underlying residual hearing loss following implantation. That work has included assessment of trauma observed during insertion trials using currently available electrode arrays [Nadol and Eddington, this vol, pp 31–49]. It has also included anatomical study of cochlear structures that are potentially vulnerable to implant-related injury. This paper reviews our findings, and those of other investigators, with attention to the implications of specific types of insertional trauma for hearing preservation.

Evaluation of Electrode Position and Insertional Trauma

Electrode arrays supplied by each of the three major implant manufacturers were used in the insertion trials. The method of microdissection for evaluation of electrode position and insertional trauma in the implanted preparations has been described in previous publications from our laboratory [5, 6]. A combination of microdissection, scanning electron microscopy, and conventional temporal bone histology was used in the studies directed toward normal cochlear morphology.

The observations discussed below are categorized according to major cochlear structures that may be susceptible to injury during implant surgery. These include the lateral wall (spiral ligament and stria vascularis), basilar membrane and cochlear duct, osseous spiral lamina and the modiolus.

Lateral Wall Trauma

Trauma to structures of the lateral cochlear wall is one of the most commonly reported types of insertional damage [7–9] and it is a significant type of injury in relation to hearing preservation. Lateral wall trauma may occur in several ways and can be due to impingement by an electrode tip or to pressure exerted by the body of the silicon carrier as it contacts the area where the basilar

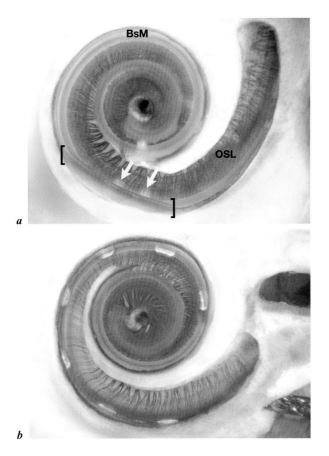

Fig. 1. a Osmium-stained inner ear dissection in which the cochlea has been opened and the angle of view is directly down on the cochlear spiral. An electrode array was inserted into scala tympani in this specimen and it lies beneath the intact osseous spiral lamina (OSL) and basilar membrane (BsM). Two of the electrode contacts, which are reflecting light, are indicated by arrows. (Other contacts are not visible in this photograph.) Although the array did not puncture the basilar membrane, it impacted the outer wall of scala tympani in such a way that the lateral wall of the cochlear duct was distorted and pushed upward in the area enclosed by brackets. The displacement of lateral wall tissues in this case can be contrasted with the specimen shown in (*b*), in which an electrode was inserted without lateral wall injury. The tissues in the basal turn are therefore in their normal configuration.

membrane joins the spiral ligament (fig. 1). Such injuries may be limited to the spiral ligament alone or may also include the basilar membrane and osseous spiral lamina [1, 7–9]. When the basilar membrane is involved, it is often torn at its attachment to the lateral wall as illustrated in figure 2, and there may, or may

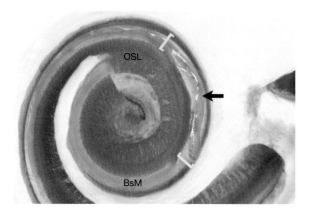

Fig. 2. Cochlear dissection illustrating an electrode insertion in which the array (arrow) has torn the basilar membrane (BsM) away from its attachment to the spiral ligament in the area enclosed by brackets. Although the basilar membrane is torn, the electrode did not deviate upward to enter the cochlear duct or scala vestibuli. The osseous spiral lamina (OSL) remains intact and was not fractured. The brownish color of the electrode is due to osmium staining of the silicon carrier. In this preparation, the apical cochlear turn was removed to provide an unobstructed view of the damaged area.

not, be penetration of the electrode into scala media. Even if the electrode does not actually enter scala media, a basilar membrane tear will open the cochlear duct, allowing intermixing of perilymph and endolymph, which has been shown in animal studies to be toxic to the stria vascularis and organ of Corti in the damaged area [10, 11]. If the electrode itself enters scala media, there will also be direct, mechanical injury of structures inside the cochlear duct, including peripheral processes of the auditory nerve, leading eventually to degeneration of spiral ganglion cells in the traumatized area [12, 13]. In more severe cases of interscalar excursion, electrodes have been found to penetrate the basilar membrane, cross through the cochlear duct, and enter scala vestibuli, where they may twist or bend back upon themselves so that the electrode tip is directed basally, toward the round window [8, 14]. As emphasized by Wardrop et al. [8], electrodes that take such an errant course in the cochlea not only produce significant trauma, but are also poorly positioned to deliver effective, frequency-appropriate stimulation because their contacts come to rest far away from the spiral ganglion cells they are intended to stimulate.

In sectioned temporal bones [7] as well as microdissected specimens, implanted electrodes have been observed to penetrate the spiral ligament beneath the basilar membrane attachment and then dissect their way between the spiral ligament and surrounding bone to reach a final position lateral to scala media (fig. 3). In these cases, the cochlear duct sometimes remains intact,

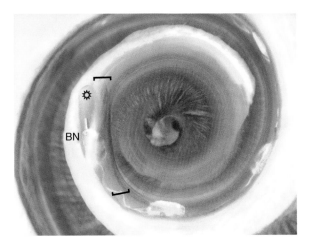

Fig. 3. An electrode insertion in which the electrode tip (open star) penetrated the spiral ligament immediately below the basilar membrane and then dissected its way between the ligament and surrounding otic capsule bone (BN) to reach a position above the basilar membrane and lateral to scala media. The electrode elevated the basilar membrane and displaced the cochlear duct medially toward the modiolus in the area enclosed by brackets.

but it is elevated and displaced medially by the electrode with attendant mechanical damage of the epithelial structures inside scala media. When the displacement is severe, Reissner's membrane will also be torn, allowing perilymph from scala vestibuli to enter the cochlear duct. In our temporal bone insertion trials, this type of injury has most often been seen with electrodes designed for relatively deep insertion and occurs when the electrode tip strikes the spiral ligament at such an angle that it pierces the connective tissue extending beneath the basilar membrane attachment zone (fig. 4).

In an effort to better understand how this type of injury occurs, we have used scanning electron microscopy to study lateral wall tissues in human temporal bones. Observations obtained to date have shown that the lower portion of the spiral ligament, under the basilar membrane, is composed of an open meshwork of connective tissue facing the perilymphatic space of scala tympani. Numerous micropores and small openings have also been observed in this location in laboratory animals and have been suggested to serve as communication routes between the perilymphatic compartment of the spiral ligament and that of scala tympani [15]. As figure 4 illustrates, this portion of the human spiral ligament has a quite delicate, irregular, porous structure. It is therefore possible that the tip of an electrode, tracking in contact with this highly textured surface might get caught in the fibrous tissue meshwork that faces scala tympani. With

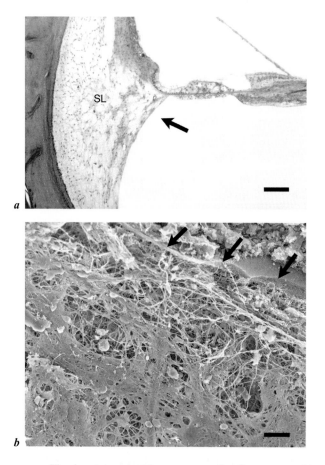

Fig. 4. *a* A temporal bone cross section from a normal human cochlea illustrating the spiral ligament (SL) and its extension below the basilar membrane. The arrow inside scala tympani indicates the angle of view for the scanning electron micrograph in (***b***), in which the surface of the spiral ligament facing scala tympani is shown. The arrows at upper right indicate the area of attachment of the basilar membrane, which was cut away to prepare this specimen. Note the porous, irregular meshwork of connective tissue at the spiral ligament surface beneath the basilar membrane attachment. Scale bar = 100 μm (***a***), 20 μm (***b***).

continued effort to advance the electrode, the tip could traumatize the surface, thereby enlarging the already existing openings, and then dissect its way into the spiral ligament immediately adjacent to the cochlear duct. This behavior would be especially likely in the upper cochlear turns where the radius of curvature of the lateral wall is such that a small-tipped electrode might strike the spiral ligament at an angle that would encourage penetration.

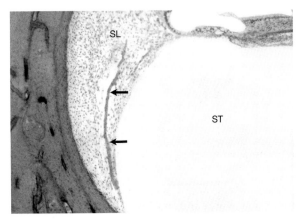

Fig. 5. Cochlear cross section showing the spiral ligament (SL) below the basilar membrane. Note the vein (arrows) coursing through the spiral ligament tissue toward the floor of scala tympani. ST = Lumen of scala tympani.

Furthermore, trauma to the spiral ligament, either by electrode penetration or compression due to pressure exerted against lateral wall tissues, is likely to damage or occlude blood vessels that provide venous drainage of the stria vascularis and spiral ligament. Those vessels course through the lower portion of the spiral ligament (fig. 5) immediately beneath the basilar membrane to reach the floor of scala tympani [16]. Interruption of the venous outflow in the lateral wall would compromise oxygen delivery to metabolically active tissues and thereby impair spiral ligament and strial function, which is essential for maintenance of the ionic composition of the cochlear fluids and the endolymphatic potential of the cochlear duct [17, 18].

Cochlear Duct/Basilar Membrane Injury

Even if an electrode does not penetrate the spiral ligament or tear the basilar membrane, it may distort and elevate these structures, as illustrated in figure 1, leading in some cases to secondary tearing of Reissner's membrane and intermixing of cochlear fluids from scala vestibuli and scala media. Upward pressure on the cochlear partition may also occlude circulation in the spiral vessel which courses on the undersurface of the basilar membrane, largely exposed to the perilymphatic space, as shown in figure 6. In addition, elevation of the cochlear duct due to upward pressure from an electrode might interfere with the normal vibrational mechanics of the basilar membrane so as to compromise the efficacy

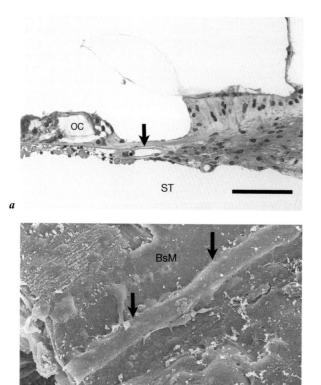

a

b

Fig. 6. *a* The cochlear cross section shows the spiral vessel (arrow) of the basilar membrane, situated in the area where the basilar membrane joins the osseous spiral lamina and facing the lumen of scala tympani (ST). OC = Organ of Corti. Scale bar = 125 μm. *b* The scanning electron micrograph shows the undersurface of the basilar membrane (BsM) and osseous spiral lamina (OSL) with the spiral vessel indicated by arrows. Note the rounded contour of the vessel, which is significantly exposed to scala tympani. Scale bar = 20 μm.

of acoustic stimulation if viable sensory epithelium is still present in the affected area of scala media.

Osseous Lamina Fracture

Our experience with implant electrode insertion into cadaveric temporal bones indicates that whenever an electrode tip becomes blocked by impingement against the spiral ligament or friction against the underside of the basilar

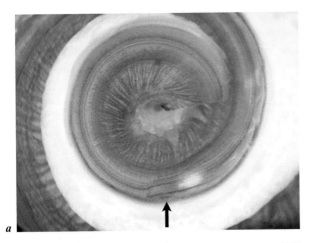

a

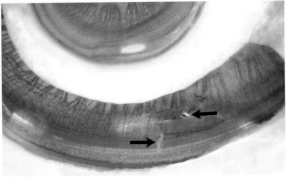

b

Fig. 7. a Cochlear dissection showing an electrode insertion in which the tip of the array met resistance in the middle turn and has elevated the basilar membrane in the area indicated by the arrow. Note the distinct bulge in the basilar membrane indicating the position of the electrode tip. Although it was displaced upward, the basilar membrane remained intact. *b* Since the tip was blocked, a continued effort to advance the electrode produced buckling in the lower basal turn, which fractured the osseous spiral lamina in the area indicated by the arrows.

membrane, any effort to further advance the electrode will produce soft tissue injury in the area of the tip. Also, if an attempt is made to advance a blocked electrode the lower portion of the array is likely to buckle upward and fracture the osseous lamina in the basal turn [19], as illustrated in figure 7. Osseous lamina fracture would, of course, sever the dendrites of spiral ganglion cells, eventually leading to ganglion cell degeneration in the affected area [1, 20].

As indicated in the discussion above, trauma involving lateral wall tissues and the basilar membrane can present a variety of potential threats to hearing conservation. In addition to the more immediate effects of lateral wall injury, there may also be longer-term consequences, such as fibrosis and osteoneogenesis which may develop due to injury of the periosteal lining of scala tympani, introduction of bone dust during cochleostomy placement or to vascular damage associated with trauma to the lateral wall or floor of scala tympani [21].

Perimodiolar Electrode Trauma to Lateral Wall and Basilar Membrane

It should be noted that lateral wall trauma is not limited to electrodes specifically designed to track in contact with the lateral wall of scala tympani, but has also been observed to occur during insertion of so-called perimodiolar electrodes engineered to place their contacts in close proximity to the modiolus. This is especially true of perimodiolar arrays that utilize space-occupying positioners, which are usually inserted with the electrode array and are intended to push the contacts toward the modiolus. Some of these devices are relatively large and can exert significant pressure against the lateral wall and basilar membrane, resulting in severe trauma, as has recently been demonstrated by Wardrop et al. [9]. Some perimodiolar arrays, not employing attached positioners, have a precurved, coiled shape that alloys the electrode to curl around the modiolus. Prior to insertion, a metal wire stylet is inserted into the silicon carrier so that the electrode is held straight as it is introduced into the cochlea. During insertion, the stylet is then progressively withdrawn so that the array regains its precurved shape and coils close to the modiolus. With this arrangement, the electrode tip tends to move away from the lateral wall during much of the insertion process. Initially, however, the electrode is straight and relatively rigid so that its tip may strike and injure the lateral wall or basilar membrane soon after it is introduced into scala tympani before the stylet is withdrawn. In addition, temporal bone insertion trials have shown that many of these electrodes do not maintain a truly perimodiolar position over their entire length (fig. 8). Particularly in the middle to upper part of the basal cochlear turn they are sometimes located against the lateral wall of scala tympani where they may injure the spiral ligament and/or basilar membrane.

Modiolar Injury

Another element of risk associated with the use of perimodiolar electrodes is the possibility of modiolar injury. If the tip of a perimodiolar electrode strikes the modiolar wall or if the body of the array is pushed into contact with the modiolus by a positioner it may easily fracture the very fragile bone covering

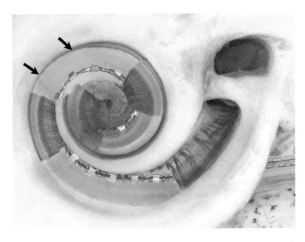

Fig. 8. A dissected specimen in which segments of the osseous spiral lamina and basilar membrane have been removed to reveal a perimodiolar electrode inserted into scala tympani. In the area indicated by the arrows the silicon carrier of the array is situated in contact with the lateral wall of scala tympani immediately below the basilar membrane attachment to the spiral ligament. In this position, such electrodes may traumatize the spiral ligament and/or basilar membrane.

the spiral ganglion (fig. 9). In addition to the possibility of acute injury of ganglion cells or their processes, the results of animal studies on chronic effects of implantation have demonstrated that even slight damage of the medial portion of the osseous spiral lamina or the modiolar wall compromises the long-term survival of ganglion cells [20].

Relative to electrodes positioned against the lateral cochlear wall, perimodiolar electrodes are likely to pose a greater hazard for inner ear damage should the need arise to explant these devices. That is due in part to the tendency for the electrode to be pulled into tighter contact with the modiolus as it is withdrawn from the cochlea. Explantation damage produced by perimodiolar electrodes has been demonstrated in a temporal bone study from Richter et al. [22]. This type of injury underscores the potential risk of modiolar trauma associated with pulling a perimodiolar electrode back at the end of the insertion procedure in order to draw contacts into close apposition to the modiolus – a maneuver previously recommended by manufacturers and which has been the subject of a recent publication [23]. Given the potential for fracture of the modiolar wall and direct mechanical injury of spiral ganglion cells, this procedure should be approached with great care.

Although it has received little attention in studies on electrode trauma, vascular damage associated with cochlear implantation represents a possible

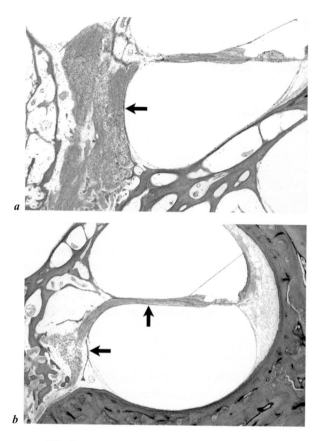

Fig. 9. Cross sections of an adult human temporal bone illustrating the very thin bone covering the cochlear nerve, spiral ganglion and osseous spiral lamina. ***a*** The middle turn region. The arrow indicates the thin bone of the modiolar wall overlying the upper portion of the spiral ganglion and cochlear nerve. ***b*** The micrograph shows the basal turn. The upper arrow indicates the osseous spiral lamina near its junction with the modiolus, and the lower arrow points out the very delicate bone covering the area of Rosenthal's canal containing the spiral ganglion.

source of functionally significant injury. This possibility has been discussed above in relation to vessels that occupy the spiral ligament and undersurface of the basilar membrane. However, blood vessels associated with the modiolus are potentially vulnerable to insertional trauma as well. Our studies of normal cochlear anatomy, using both pediatric and adult temporal bones, have shown that veins located near the modiolar wall often have little or no bony covering and are thus essentially exposed to the perilymphatic space of scala tympani. As illustrated in figure 10, this is true of vessels that course on the side of the

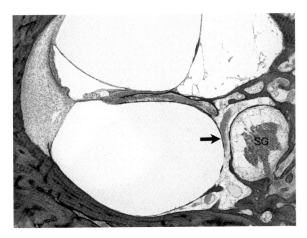

Fig. 10. A modiolar cross section showing a vein (arrow) located on the side of the modiolus and covered only by a thin layer of bone. This blood vessel is quite similar to one illustrated in the dissected specimen shown in figure 11. SG = Spiral ganglion.

modiolus, connecting the anterior spiral vein located near the root of the osseous lamina with the larger posterior spiral vein which takes a spiral course in the area where the modiolus meets the floor of scala tympani. The cochlear dissection shown in figure 11 demonstrates that the posterior spiral vein may be largely exposed at the base of the modiolar wall and is therefore susceptible to electrode-induced trauma. This vein provides the major venous outflow for the cochlea and receives tributaries from the osseous lamina, the modiolus, and veins distributed on the floor of scala tympani, which receive venous blood from lateral wall structures. Therefore, injury of this vessel could potentially compromise circulation to a large part of the cochlea.

Trauma Associated with Cochleostomy Placement

Finally, it should be noted that cochlear injury associated with placement of a cochleostomy represents yet another aspect of insertional trauma. Variable damage to the periosteal lining of scala tympani and blood vessels associated with the area is of course unavoidable during cochleostomy placement. Bone dust, which may contribute to development of fibrosis and osteoneogenesis, is also frequently intro-duced into the perilymphatic space during the drilling procedure. The extent of sur-gical injury, loss of perilymph and introduction of bone dust can be limited to some degree by use of the so-called 'soft surgery' technique [24] in which the otic capsule bone is removed to the point of exposing the periosteal lining of scala tympani, but

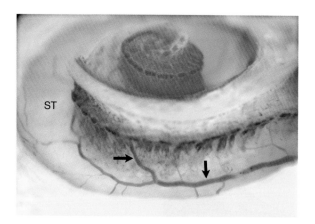

Fig. 11. Cochlear dissection showing veins associated with the modiolus. In this preparation the osseous spiral lamina and basilar membrane have been removed to provide a view of the floor of scala tympani and modiolar wall. The specimen has been stained with osmium tetroxide; however, no bone or periosteum has been removed in the areas where the superficially located blood vessels are seen. The horizontal arrow indicates a vein coursing down the modiolar wall to join the posterior spiral vein (downward-pointing arrow) which lies at the junction of the modiolar wall with the floor of scala tympani (ST).

the periostium is not incised until immediately before electrode insertion. Application of suction in the area of the cochleostomy is also carefully avoided.

In most cases, there is restricted visibility of the cochlear promontory and round window margin via a facial recess opening when the posterior tympanotomy approach is used for electrode insertion. The accuracy of placement and angulation of a cochleostomy anterior to the round window can therefore be somewhat problematic and the margin of error is quite small. If the cochleostomy is placed too high on the promontory, injury is likely to occur at the area of attachment of the basilar membrane to the spiral ligament, which may violate the cochlear duct and fracture the osseous spiral lamina. Trauma associated with cochleostomy placement has been noted in previous temporal bone studies [25] and has been observed in our laboratory as well (fig. 12). Also, the position and angulation of the cochleostomy may significantly affect the behavior of an electrode as it is introduced into scala tympani, occasionally leading to basilar membrane damage or contact by the electrode against the modiolar wall. Moreover, the size of the cochleostomy opening may be a factor. If the cochleostomy is large relative to the diameter of the electrode, a very flexible array will have greater freedom of movement during insertion, so that if the tip meets resistance there is increased likelihood that the electrode will buckle in the lower base and fracture the osseous spiral lamina. Various aspects of

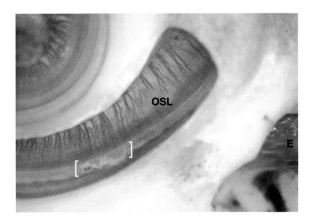

Fig. 12. Dissected specimen illustrating basilar membrane damage (area enclosed by brackets) that occurred during drilling of a cochleostomy. The cochleostomy opening was placed somewhat too high on the promontory so that the drill bit produced a tear in the basilar membrane. E = A portion of the electrode array situated just outside the cochleostomy entrance; OSL = osseous spiral lamina.

cochleostomy placement are therefore important for avoiding injury and assuring successful electrode insertion.

Modifications in Electrode Design

As discussed above, the lateral wall of the cochlea and the modiolus are both highly vulnerable to insertional trauma. It may therefore be that electrode arrays designed to occupy the mid-portion of scala tympani and thereby minimize contact with either the lateral or medial walls of the perilymphatic space during insertion will be advantageous in terms of avoiding injury. As stressed by Leake and Rebscher [1], restricting the vertical flexibility of electrodes so that they are less likely to undergo upward defection toward the basilar membrane or osseous lamina is also an important design feature that will reduce the incidence of trauma. This can be achieved by incorporating a central rib in the silicon carrier or by arranging the contact wiring in such a way that the array is more flexible in the medial-lateral plane than in the vertical plane. Other features such as modifications of tip shape and electrode curvature to help avoid spiral ligament penetration by electrodes intended to track the lateral wall may be beneficial as well. For selected patients who retain significant levels of low-frequency hearing and who are likely to benefit from electro-acoustic stimulation technology, use of a short electrode array as advocated by Gantz et al. [2] may offer important advantages.

Such an electrode, confined to the base of the cochlea and occupying the middle of scala tympani would permit electrical stimulation of high-frequency neural elements with significantly reduced potential for insertional trauma, thereby helping to ensure that neurosensory stuctures in the upper portion of the cochlea remain viable and functionally responsive to acoustic stimulation.

Implications for Surgical Technique

Careful analysis of insertional trauma has implications for surgical technique as well as for electrode design. Surgeons must stop the insertion process when resistance to insertion is first encountered to prevent the electrode tip from penetrating cochlear soft tissues and to avoid buckling of the basal portion of the electrode, which may fracture the osseous spiral lamina. 'Pulling back' the electrode in order to bring the contacts into closer proximity to the modiolus must be done with caution, lest the tip of the electrode be dragged retrograde over the delicate surface of the modiolus. Cochleostomies need to be carefully placed to reduce the likelihood of injury to the spiral ligament, organ of Corti, basilar membrane and osseous spiral lamina.

Alternative Insertion Procedures

There has been a recent revival of interest in using the round window membrane itself as the insertion point for electrodes placed in scala tympani, and this approach has potential advantages for minimizing insertional injury. The round window was abandoned as a portal of access to scala tympani in the early years of cochlear implantation because better visualization of scala tympani is obtained with a separate cochleostomy made anterior to the round window niche. The standard promontory cochleostomy, however, is associated with significant acoustic trauma, loss of perilymph and potentially allows bone dust to enter scala tympani. An insertion directly through the round window membrane avoids these causes of hearing loss and, therefore, has theoretical appeal, especially when hearing conservation is the goal.

Round Window Insertion, Surgical Considerations

The round window membrane is a thin, soft tissue barrier between scala tympani and the middle ear which offers the possibility to pass an electrode from the middle ear into scala tympani without any drilling at all. The membrane, however, is recessed within the round window niche. It is partially (and often completely) hidden from view when looking directly down the external auditory canal and, to a lesser extent, when looking through the facial recess. Occasionally, some part of the round window membrane (but rarely more than one third) can be visualized through a facial recess approach, if the facial recess is extended inferiorly as far as possible. A full view of the round window membrane can only be obtained by drilling off both the anterior-inferior and posterior lips of the round window niche. Posteriorly, the round window membrane is somewhat horizontal and separated from the osseous spiral lamina by less than 1 mm. Opening the posterior/superior half of the round window membrane does not provide surgically useful access to scala tympani and previous investigators have regularly emphasized that the posterior/superior portion of the round window membrane does not need to be well visualized to insert an electrode into scala tympani.

The anterior/inferior half of the round window, where the membrane is nearly vertical can be well visualized by removing only the anterior/inferior lip of the niche. The amount of drilling required to expose the round window membrane is significantly less than that required to perform a classic cochleostomy over the mid portion of the promontory, where bone overlying scala tympani is thickest. However, removing the anterior/inferior portion of the round window membrane, while providing adequate access for insertion of an electrode array, does not provide a 'good view' of scala tympani. If a clear view of scala tympani is to be obtained, then either the crista semilunaris at the medial inferior portion of the round window niche or the anterior/inferior portion of the round window niche needs to be removed. However, bone removal in this area can be minimal. Reduction in the amount of drilling should reduce the risk of acoustic trauma and minimize the introduction of bone dust into scala tympani.

Because an electrode inserted through the round window enters scala tympani more basally than would be the case when using a standard cochleostomy, it is possible that more basally located neural elements would become available for stimulation than with a traditional promontory cochleostomy insertion. Whether or not this would provide an advantage for speech perception (especially in noise) remains unclear. The issue concerns not only potential stimulation of residual dendrites in the most basal portion of the cochlea, but also the possibility that access to the modiolus in this area would permit more localized stimulation of a population of spiral ganglion cells that may otherwise be inaccessible.

An additional positive feature of round window insertion is that it may be possible to seal the tissues around the electrode more quickly, and more completely than with a classic promontory cochleostomy. However, more effective healing of a round window membrane cochleostomy has not been proven.

Finally, it is hoped that electrode insertion through an incision in the round window membrane might reduce the loss of perilymph. In a perfect dissection it is possible to expose the endosteum of scala tympani without violating it during the performance of a classic promontory cochleostomy. However, it is a practical reality that this is not always achieved in the operating room. Even with great care, the drill bit frequently tears or perforates the endosteum of scala tympani despite the surgeon's best efforts to prevent it from doing so. However, If the volume of perilymph within scala tympani is in fact preserved, care must be given during electrode insertion to avoid hydrodynamic fluid displacement that may injure the basilar membrane and/or the organ of Corti. Presumably very slow insertions with controlled outflow of perilymph through the round window membrane incision would be necessary.

Possible Difficulties with Round Window Insertion

In spite of its potential advantages, there are a number of technical difficulties and possible disadvantages associated with round window membrane insertion. The round window membrane is concave, with its deepest portion lying within the medial portions of scala tympani. Consequently, its upper portion is nearly horizontal and lies close to the osseous spiral lamina. At its closest point, it approaches to within 0.1 mm of the osseous spiral lamina and, therefore, great care must be taken when inserting an electrode through the round window membrane to avoid injury to the osseous spiral lamina. However, laboratory data suggest that simple fracture of the osseous spiral lamina would produce only discreet loss of spiral ganglion cells, subserving the frequency range of only the traumatized area. More severe trauma involving penetration of scala media would allow intermixing of perilymph and endolymph which might cause more widespread loss of residual hearing, since perilymph is toxic to hair cells.

Because of the proximity of the osseous spiral lamina, the presence of the crista semilunaris and the inferior/anterior direction of scala tympani, an electrode passing through the round window membrane would require a very careful angle of insertion. However, our laboratory studies have shown that it is possible to insert a straight electrode directly into the scala tympani using a round window membrane approach. These studies have also demonstrated that such an insertion must be done so that the electrode passes in a 'posterior/superior' to 'anterior/inferior' direction.

Middle ear mucosa frequently covers the round window niche or membrane. Such a 'false' round window membrane must be distinguished from the round window membrane itself. Moreover, the bony anatomy of the round window niche is notoriously variable, and the surgeon attempting a round window membrane insertion must be familiar with these variations if removal of the anterior/inferior portion of the round window niche is to be accomplished with minimal drilling and minimal trauma.

If the purpose of utilizing a round window membrane approach is conservation of hearing, then the physiologic function of the round window membrane must be retained. The round window membrane serves as a relief valve, allowing displacement of perilymph as the stapedial footplate moves inward. Perilymph, like water, is noncompressible and downward movement of the footplate cannot produce a traveling wave unless fluid displacement can be accommodated. However, electrode insertion via the round window is unlikely to severely jeopardize round window membrane function. In fact, the work of the Warsaw group under Henryk Skarzynski has shown that even the relatively thick Med-El Combi 40+ electrode can be passed through the round window membrane up to 20 mm into scala tympani without affecting residual hearing.

Endoscopically Assisted Round Window Insertion

We are currently performing laboratory studies on endoscopically assisted round window membrane insertions. It is possible to fully visualize the round window membrane with a 30° endoscope passed through the external auditory canal. Obviously, this requires a tympanomeatal flap in addition to a facial recess approach. However, we have verified that it is possible to visualize the entire round window membrane in this fashion without removing any bone, to incise the round window membrane, and then to pass an electrode through it and fully insert it into scala tympani. These observations are encouraging. It is hoped that it will eventually be possible to reliably, routinely, and safely pass an electrode into scala tympani without any removal of bone.

References

1   Leake PA, Rebscher SJ: Anatomical considerations and long-term effects of electrical stimulation; in Zeng FG, Popper AN, Fay RR (eds): Cochlear Implants, Auditory Prostheses and Electrical Hearing. Springer Handbook of Auditory Research. New York, Springer, 2004, vol 20, pp 100–148.
2   Gantz BJ, Turner C, Gfeller KE, Lowder MW: Preservation of hearing in cochlear implant surgery: advantages of combined electrical and acoustical speech processing. Laryngoscope 2005;115:796–802.
3   Hodges AV, Schloffman J, Balkany T: Conservation of residual hearing with cochlear implantation. Am J Otol 1997;18:179–183.
4   Skarzynski H, Lorens A, D'Haese P, Walkowiak A, Piotrowska A, Sliwa L, Anderson I: Preservation of residual hearing in children and post-lingually deafened adults after cochlear implantation: an initial study. ORL 2002;64:247–253.
5   Wright CG, Roland PS: Temporal bone microdissection for anatomic study of cochlear implant electrodes. Cochlear Implants Int 2005;6:159–168.

6 Wright CG, Roland PS, Kuzma J: Advanced Bionics Thin Lateral and Helix II electrodes: a temporal bone study. Laryngoscope 2005;115:2046–2050.

7 Nadol JB, Shiao JY, Burgess BJ, Ketten DR, Eddington DK, Gantz BJ, Kos I, Montandon P, Coker NJ, Roland JT, Shallop JK: Histopathology of cochlear implants in humans. Ann Otol Rhinol Laryngol 2001;110:883–891.

8 Wardrop P, Whinney D, Rebscher SJ, Roland TJ, Luxford W, Leak PA: A temporal bone study of insertion trauma and intracochlear position of cochlear implant electrodes. I. Comparison of Nucleus banded and Nucleus Contour electrodes. Hear Res 2005;203:54–67.

9 Wardrop P, Whinney D, Rebscher SJ, Luxford W, Leake P: A temporal bone study of insertion trauma and intracochlear position of cochlear implant electrodes. II. Comparison of Spiral Clarion and HiFocus II electrodes. Hear Res 2005;203:68–79.

10 Duvall AJ, Rhodes VT: Ultrastucture of the organ of Corti following intermixing of fluids. Ann Otol Rhinol Laryngol 1967;76:688–708.

11 Shaddock LC, Wright CG, Hamernik R: A morphometric study of microvascular pathology following experimental rupture of Reissner's membrane. Hear Res 1985;20:119–129.

12 Spoendlin H: Factors inducing retrograde degeneration of the cochlear nerve. Ann Otol Rhinol Laryngol 1984;93:76–82.

13 Sugawara M, Corfas G, Liberman MC: Influence of supporting cells on neuronal degeneration after hair cell loss. J Assoc Res Otolaryngol 2005;6:136–147.

14 Ketten DR, Skinner MW, Wang, GE, Vannier MW, Gates GA, Neely JG: In vivo measures of cochlear length and insertion depth of Nucleus cochlear implant electrode arrays. Ann Otol Rhinol Laryngol 1998;107:1–16.

15 Lim D: Surface ultrastructure of the cochlear perilymphatic space. J Laryngol Otol 1970;84: 413–428.

16 Axelsson A: The vascular anatomy of the cochlea in the guinea pig and in man. Acta Otolaryngol 1968;243(suppl):1–134.

17 Spicer SS, Schulte B: Differentiation of inner ear fibrocytes according to their ion transport related activity. Hear Res 1991;56:53–64.

18 Wangemann P, Liu J, Marcus DC: Ion transport mechanisms responsible for K^+ secretion and the transepithelial voltage across marginal cells of stria vascularis in vitro. Hear Res 1995;84:19–29.

19 Gstoettner W, Plenk H, Franz P, Hamzavi J, Baumgartner W, Czerny C, Ehrenberger K: Cochlear implant deep electrode insertion: extent of insertional trauma. Acta Otolaryngol 1997;117: 274–277.

20 Leake PA, Hradek GT, Snyder RL: Chronic electrical stimulation by a cochlear implant promotes survival of spiral ganglion neurons in neonatally deafened cats. J Comp Neurol 1999;412: 543–562.

21 Nadol JB: Patterns of neural degeneration in the human cochlea and auditory nerve: implications for cochlear implantation. Otolaryngol Head Neck Surg 1997;117:220–228.

22 Richter B, Jaekel K, Aschendorff A, Marangos N, Laszig R: Cochlear structures after implantation of a perimodiolar electrode array. Laryngoscope 2001;111:837–842.

23 Todt I, Basta D, Eisenschenk A, Ernst A: The 'pull-back' technique for Nucleus 24 perimodiolar electrode insertion. Otolaryngol Head Neck Surg 2005;132:751–754.

24 Lehnhardt E: Intracochlear placement of cochlear implant electrodes in soft surgery technique. HNO 1993;41:356–359.

25 Adunka O, Kiefer J, Unkelbach MH, Lehnert T: Development and evaluation of an improved cochlear implant electrode design for electric acoustic stimulation. Laryngoscope 2004;114:1237–1241.

Charles G. Wright, PhD
Callier Center for Communication Disorders
1966 Inwood Road
Dallas, TX 75235 (USA)
Tel. +1 214 905 3117, Fax +1 214 905 3053, E-Mail cgwrigh@Utdallas.edu

Møller AR (ed): Cochlear and Brainstem Implants.
Adv Otorhinolaryngol. Basel, Karger, 2006, vol 64, pp 31–49

....

Histopathology of the Inner Ear Relevant to Cochlear Implantation

Joseph B. Nadol Jr.[a,b], *Donald K. Eddington*[a,c,d]

[a]Department of Otology and Laryngology, Harvard Medical School, [b]Department of Otolaryngology, [c]Cochlear Implant Research Laboratory, Massachusetts Eye and Ear Infirmary, [d]Research Laboratory of Electronics, Massachusetts Institute of Technology, Boston, Mass., USA

Abstract

The most common forms of severe hearing loss and deafness are related to morphological changes in the cochlea. Many individuals with such forms of hearing disorders have received cochlear implants. It has been assumed that preservation of spiral ganglion cells is important for success of cochlear implants. Preservation of ganglion cells is negatively correlated with the duration of the hearing loss. It has, however, not been possible to reveal a relationship between the degree of survival of spiral ganglion cells and performance of cochlear implants. It is important to understand the histopathological changes that follow cochlear implantation. Insertion of cochlear implants may cause trauma to the basilar membrane, the spiral lamina, and the spiral ligament. Rupture of the basilar membrane may occur. Over time, new bone forms at the cochleostomy and along the implant track. Further investigation is necessary to evaluate the causes of variability of behavioral measures of performance.

Copyright © 2006 S. Karger AG, Basel

The wide variability of success as measured by open set speech discrimination in individual patients who have undergone cochlear implantation has added renewed relevance to the histopathology of severe to profound deafness. In addition, as temporal bones from individuals who in life had undergone cochlear implantation become available, study of the pathologic changes induced by cochlear implantation and correlation of the success of implantation with histopathology have become possible [Roland and Wright, this vol, pp 11–30]. This paper reviews the pertinent histopathology of severe to profound deafness in the human and what has been learned from study of temporal bones from patients who underwent cochlear implantation during life.

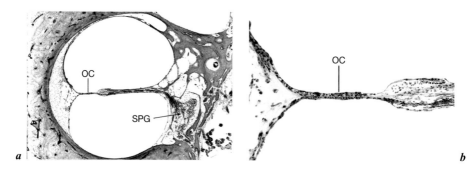

Fig. 1. Cochlear hair cells from a 65-year-old man with cochleosaccular dysplasia and cataracts, a disorder inherited as an autosomal dominant trait, who suffered a progressive bilateral sensorineural hearing loss beginning at age 26. His hearing loss was severe to profound by age 58. The principal correlate of the sensorineural hearing loss was total loss of the organ of Corti (OC) throughout the cochlea. Although the neuronal population was reduced, there were spiral ganglion cells (SPG) throughout the cochlea. *a* Basal turn. *b* High power of the region normally occupied by the organ of Corti.

Histopathology of Deafness in Humans

Although some cases of central deafness have been described [1] and evidence that cognitive defects play a role in hearing loss of the aged has accrued [2], the most important correlates of severe to profound deafness in the human are various forms of degeneration of the inner ear. Evidence for this includes histopathology of the ear [3, 4], which has been at least in part corroborated by modern imaging of the auditory cortex [5]. Although originally designed for the study of human presbycusis [6], the categorization of subtypes of hearing disorders by specific cell and tissue targets may be applied more generally to other etiologies of deafness [7, 8]. The principal peripheral cellular targets are auditory hair cells (fig. 1), the stria vascularis (fig. 2) and first order cochlear neurons (fig. 3). More recently, the possible role of dysfunction of the lateral cochlear wall in the causation of sensorineural loss has been identified [8–11].

Degeneration of Spiral Ganglion Cells and Their Processes

Although word recognition scores range widely in all published series of cochlear implantation [12, 13; see also Geers, this vol, pp 50–65], the histopathologic correlates of success are as yet not completely known. However, it is generally assumed that the residual spiral ganglion cell population in the deaf ear is a critical factor in determining the success of implantation [14, 15].

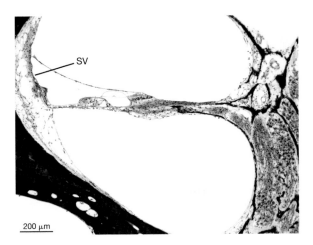

Fig. 2. Stria vascularis in a 94-year-old woman who suffered a bilateral progressive sensorineural hearing loss beginning at approximately 30 years of age. The family history suggested a genetic etiology. An audiogram at age 89 demonstrated bilateral 80–100 dB sensorineural loss. There was severe atrophy of the stria vascularis (SV) in all turns, partial loss of outer hair cells, and moderate loss of cochlear neurons in the basal turn. The principal histopathologic correlate of the flat sensorineural hearing loss audiometric pattern was severe atrophy of the stria vascularis.

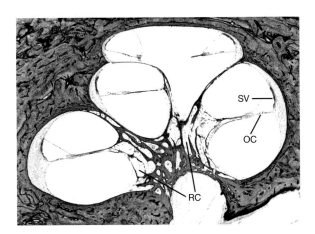

Fig. 3. Cochlear degeneration in a 41-year-old woman who suffered a sudden sensorineural hearing loss in her right ear at the age of 18 years. Audiometry demonstrated a profound loss in the right ear. Throughout the cochlea there was a total loss of spiral ganglion cells in Rosenthal's canal (RC), whereas the organ of Corti (OC) and stria vascularis (SV) were normal.

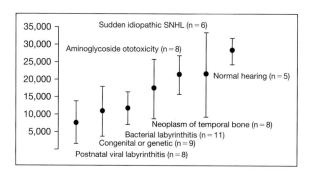

Fig. 4. Means and standard deviations of spiral ganglion cell counts in six most common diagnostic categories of etiologies of hearing loss and in 5 individuals with normal hearing. Reprinted with permission from Nadol et al. [4].

Both primary and secondary degeneration of the spiral ganglion cells occur and are more common in the basal as compared to the apical half of the cochlea [16]. Although all the factors that determine degree and speed of secondary degeneration of spiral ganglion cells in the human are unknown, it is most severe when both inner hair cells [17] and outer hair cells are missing [16], and when there has been degeneration of cochlear supporting [18], loss of pillar and Deiter cells [19] or injury of the peripheral terminal processes of cochlear neurons [20]. Primary degeneration of the spiral ganglion cell and its processes may occur with no obvious neuroepithelial changes in such disorders as presbycusis [6], sudden deafness [21], Friedrick's ataxia [22], Usher's syndrome [23] and some genetically determined disorders [24] such as in the deaf white cat.

In 93 temporal bones from 66 patients who during life had a documented profound sensorineural hearing loss [4], the duration of hearing loss and duration of profound deafness were found to be negatively correlated with residual spiral ganglion cell count. The main determinant of the total spiral ganglion cell count in this study was the cause of deafness (fig. 4). These findings are consistent with previous studies [25, 26], although other authors have found no correlation between residual spiral ganglion cell count and cause of deafness [3]. Although there is significant intersubject variation of spiral ganglion cell counts within diagnostic categories, it is rare for there to be total spiral ganglion counts less than 10,000 [3, 4].

Because of the variability of spiral ganglion cell counts determined by diagnosis, age, and duration of deafness, it is attractive to search for clinical markers such as the diameter of the eighth nerve on MRI imaging that might correlate with residual spiral ganglion cell count. In a temporal bone study of 42 patients who in life were profoundly deaf and would have been candidates for cochlear

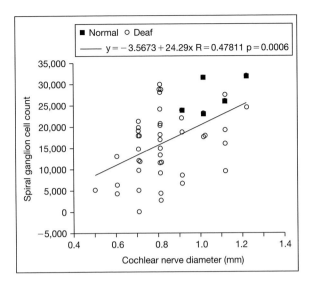

Fig. 5. Scatter plot demonstrating the correlation between the spiral ganglion cell count and diameter of the cochlear nerve. Reprinted with permission from Nadol and Xu [27].

implantation and in 5 patients with normal hearing, the maximum diameter of the cochlear, vestibular, and eighth cranial nerves were measured histologically. Although the maximum diameters were significantly smaller in the deaf population as compared to the normal hearing controls, only 25% of the variance of the spiral ganglion cell count was predicted by the maximum diameter of the eighth nerve (fig. 5). Therefore, although imaging studies may be helpful in predicting residual spiral ganglion cell counts, the precision is low [27].

*Specific Causes of Deafness of Special Relevance to
Cochlear Implantation*

Bacterial Labyrinthitis
Patients deafened by bacterial meningitis are frequent candidates for cochlear implantation. However, new bone formation within the cochlea, or labyrinthitis ossificans, is a common finding in such individuals [28, 29] (fig. 6). The presence of labyrinthitis ossificans is recognizable on imaging of the temporal bone, and creates a mechanical impediment to implantation. In addition, there is a significant negative correlation between percent bony occlusion and the percent of normal spiral ganglion cell counts [30, 31] (fig. 7). In all cases in which the segmental and total bony occlusion was less than 10%, there was at

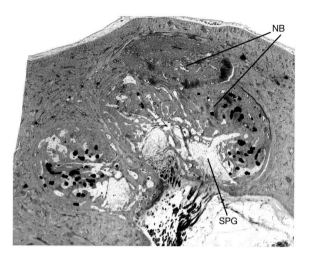

Fig. 6. Ossification of the cochlea in a 5-year-old boy who became profoundly and bilaterally deaf as a consequence of streptococcal meningitis at the age of 18 months. Two months following recovery from meningitis, a CT of the temporal bone showed no evidence of labyrinthitis ossificans. However, a repeat CT scan done 2 months thereafter showed new bone growth in both cochleae, worse on the right side. In this right ear, the cochlea is largely replaced by new bone (NB) in all turns. Although there is no recognizable organ of Corti, there were residual spiral ganglion cells (SPG) with a total spiral ganglion cell count of 10,900.

least 30% of the age-matched normal segmental and total spiral ganglion cell densities. However, even in cases with severe bony occlusion, significant numbers of spiral ganglion cells survive. Total absence of spiral ganglion cells was not found in any specimen with labyrinthitis ossificans secondary to bacterial meningitis.

Genetically Determined Sensorineural Hearing Loss
Postnatal Progressive Deafness
Similar to other causes of deafness, the histopathologic correlates of genetically determined postnatal progressive sensorineural loss are degeneration of various elements of the inner ear. Bony malformation of the cochlea is relatively uncommon. Usher's syndrome and DFNA-9 are presented as examples of syndromic and nonsyndromic causes of postnatal, progressive, sensorineural hearing loss.

Usher's Syndrome
Usher's syndrome is the most common cause of autosomal recessive pattern of syndromic deafness. There are three distinguishable subtypes of Usher's

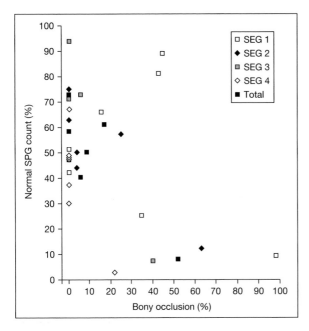

Fig. 7. A scatter plot demonstrating the correlation of percent normal spiral ganglion cell count by segment and total spiral ganglion cell count with the percentage of bony occlusion of the cochlear duct in six cases of meningogenic labyrinthitis. Reprinted with permission from Nadol and Hsu [30].

syndrome (I, II, III) which are differentiated on the basis of onset and degree of hearing impairment, and vestibular dysfunction. Thus, in Usher's syndrome type I there is congenital, severe to profound, sensorineural loss and vestibular dysfunction, whereas in Usher's syndrome type II there is a congenital hearing loss without deafness and normal vestibular function. In Usher's syndrome type III, there is a progressive loss of hearing and progressive vestibulopathy.

There are at least seven different gene mutations for Usher's syndrome type I and at least four for Usher's type II. The histopathology of the inner ear in Usher's syndrome in all reported cases of all types includes degeneration of hair cells of the organ of Corti and spiral ganglion cells [23, 32–34] (fig. 8).

DFNA-9

DFNA-9 is an autosomal dominantly inherited disorder, which produces adult onset sensorineural loss. The molecular genetic basis of this disorder has been demonstrated [35] as a missense mutation in the cochlear gene COCH. This disorder is of interest not only because its molecular genetics are understood, but

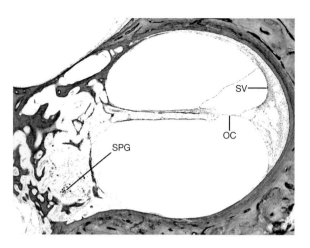

Fig. 8. This 82-year-old woman suffered profound congenital deafness as a consequence of Usher's syndrome type I. The histopathologic correlate of this deafness included atrophy of the stria vascularis (SV), total loss of the organ of Corti (OC), and the severe loss of spiral ganglion cells (SPG). However, there was a residual spiral ganglion cell count of 6,776, approximately 40% of age-matched controls.

also because of unique histopathology [36] (fig. 9). The histopathologic correlate of profound sensorineural loss includes marked degeneration of the spiral ligament and severe degeneration of spiral ganglion cells. Specifically, the dendritic processes of spiral ganglion cells, normally seen in the osseous spiral lamina, are missing and replaced by an eosinophilic acellular material, whereas the spiral ganglion cells do remain, albeit in reduced numbers. This is of particular interest because patients with this disorder who have undergone cochlear implantation are in general good implant users [pers. obs.], suggesting that peripheral processes (dendrites) of spiral ganglion cells are not necessary for neural stimulation using a cochlear implant.

Congenital Deafness

Approximately 25% of congenitally deaf individuals have a recognizable malformation of the otic capsule [37]. These abnormalities range from minor defects to total aplasia of the cochlea. These malformations create special challenges to successful implantation including widely patent communications between the spinal fluid space and perilymphatic scalae via a malformed cribrose area, potentially causing a cerebrospinal fluid leak; abnormal juxtaposition of the vestibular apparatus to the cochlea, increasing the possibility of unintended stimulation of vestibular neurons by a cochlear implant; difficult

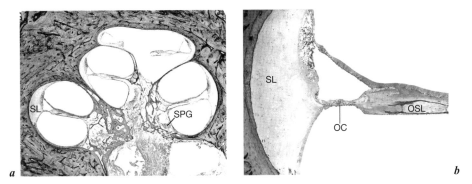

Fig. 9. This 59-year-old woman suffered a progressive bilateral sensorineural loss starting at the age of 21 years secondary to an autosomal dominant disorder (DFNA-9). An audiogram at age 50 years demonstrated a severe to profound sensorineural hearing loss in this right ear, with 0% speech discrimination. Pathologic study demonstrated eosinophilic extracellular material infiltrating the spiral ligament (SL) and the osseous spiral lamina (OSL). Although there were residual spiral ganglion cells (SPG) in Rosenthal's canal, there was total atrophy of the peripheral dendrites in the OSL. Hair cells in the organ of Corti (OC) were present in all three turns of the cochlea. *a* Midmodiolar section. *b* Higher power of basal turn (line up *b* with *a*).

access for cochlear implantation due to absence of the round window and/or malpositioned facial nerve, and decreased and anomalously located spiral ganglion cells in a rudimentary modiolus and Rosenthal's canal (fig. 10).

In summary, except in rare cases, the histopathology of severe to profound deafness in the human is located primarily in the inner ear. It is rare for there to be total degeneration of the spiral ganglion cells, although the distribution and total number of these cells vary widely.

Histopathologic Changes in the Cochlea Induced by Cochlear Implantation

The insertion of a cochlear implant electrode array causes a varying amount of immediate trauma and also results in delayed effects.

Immediate Trauma Caused by Cochlear Implants

Depending upon the location and size of the cochleostomy, significant trauma may occur to the basilar membrane and osseous spiral lamina (figs. 11, 12). Displacement of the basilar membrane or fracture-dislocation of the osseous spiral

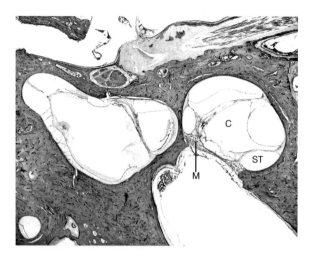

Fig. 10. This 85-year-old woman suffered congenital deafness secondary to severe dysplasia of the bony cochlea and vestibular system. There were approximately one to half turns in the rudimentary cochlea (C). There were no hair cells. The modiolus (M) was rudimentary. There were, however, a few spiral ganglion cells remaining. The scala tympani (ST) of the basal turn was markedly reduced in size.

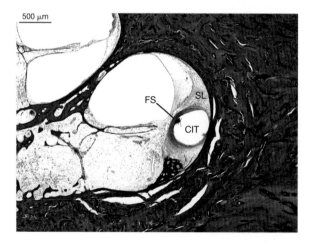

Fig. 11. Example of acute trauma caused by cochlear implantation in a 91-year-old man with bilateral progressive and profound sensorineural hearing loss who underwent cochlear implantation of the left ear 11 years prior to death. The cochlear implant track (CIT) is visible. In this basal turn, the implant array had penetrated the spiral ligament (SL) and was surrounded by a fibrous sheath (FS).

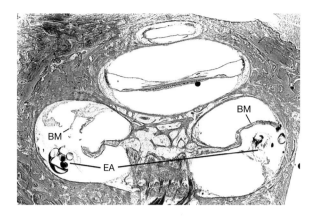

Fig. 12. Acute trauma from cochlear implantation in a 62-year-old woman who suffered a progressive loss of hearing and profound deafness bilaterally as a consequence of aminoglycoside ototoxicity 5 years prior to implantation. In her implanted right ear, the electrode array (EA) has been maintained in situ. There is fracture-dislocation of the basilar membrane (BM) on the left approximately 11 mm from the round window membrane, and displacement of the basilar membrane (BM) on the right, approximately 18 mm from the round window membrane by the electrode array.

lamina is not uncommon [38; see also Roland and Wright, this vol, pp 11–30]. Occasionally, a rupture of the basilar membrane may occur with the passage of a cochlear implant from scala tympani into scala vestibuli.

Damage to the lateral cochlear wall, particularly in the ascending limb of the basal turn, may occur.

Delayed Effects Induced by Cochlear Implantation

New bone formation is a universal finding, particularly near the cochleostomy site following cochlear implantation [38]. A fibrous tissue sheath surrounds the implant electrode within the middle ear and also within the inner ear. New bone formation may extend along the implantation track to a variable length and sometimes may extend apical to the end of the implant array. For examples of delayed effects induced by cochlear implantation, see figures 13, 14.

Effect on Spiral Ganglion Cells

In a study of 11 cochleae from patients who in life had undergone cochlear implantation and in whom the contralateral, nonimplanted ear was available, the mean spiral ganglion cell count for the implanted and nonimplanted ears were not significantly different in the most basal three of four segments of the

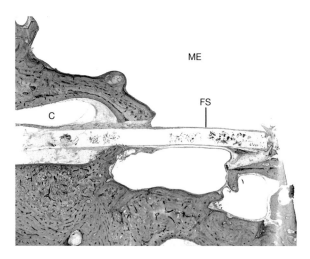

Fig. 13. Delayed effect of cochlear implantation in a 74-year-old man who underwent right cochlear implantation 12 years before death for rehabilitation of a progressive and profound sensorineural hearing loss. A dense fibrous sheath (FS) is present, not only within the cochlea (C), but also extends at least several millimeters into the middle ear (ME).

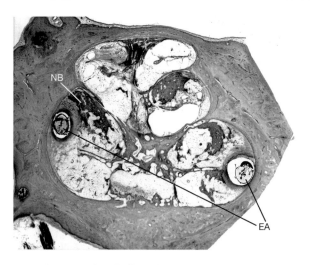

Fig. 14. Delayed effect of cochlear implantation in a 64-year-old woman who suffered a profound bilateral sensorineural hearing loss secondary to cochleosaccular degeneration. A CT scan of the inner ear done 10 years prior to death showed no abnormality of the cochlea. Three months later, she underwent a left cochlear implant with no insertional difficulties. In the right ear, there was evidence of cochlear saccular degeneration, but no evidence of new bone formation. However, in the left ear there was new bone (NB) formation surrounding the electrode array (EA) in the scala vestibuli and extending apical to it. Based on the otologic history, preoperative CT scan, and comparison with the opposite temporal bone, this new bone formation was judged to be a consequence of the cochlear implantation.

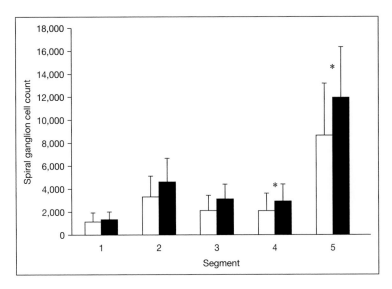

Fig. 15. Mean segmental and total spiral ganglion cell counts in implanted (□) and nonimplanted (■) cochleae in 11 patients. Vertical bars = 1 SD, *p < 0.01. Reprinted with permission from Khan et al. [39].

cochlea. However, a modest decrease in spiral ganglion cell count was found in the most apical segment and in the total spiral ganglion cell count [39] (fig. 15). In addition, there was no relationship between the interaural difference in spiral ganglion cell counts and duration of implantation, suggesting that a progressive loss of spiral ganglion cells after implantation did not occur. The fact that there was no statistical difference in the basal three segments of the cochlea where the implanted electrode could possibly cause direct physical trauma to the osseous spiral lamina or dendritic processes of the spiral ganglion cells suggests that any differences in spiral ganglion cell count were not due to implantation trauma.

A lack of significant difference in spiral ganglion cell counts seen in human subjects is consistent with findings in experimental animals [40], and in previous reports in human subjects [41–43].

Tissue Seal at Cochleostomy Site

Bacterial meningitis has been reported as an infrequent delayed complication of cochlear implantation using a variety of electrode designs [44–46]. The cause of meningitis in cochlear implant recipients is not fully understood. Predisposing factors may include a previous history of meningitis, congenital anomalies of the cochlea, age less than 5 years, otitis media, immunodeficiency states or surgical technique. The possibility of an open communication between the middle and inner ears has been raised as another possible cause [47].

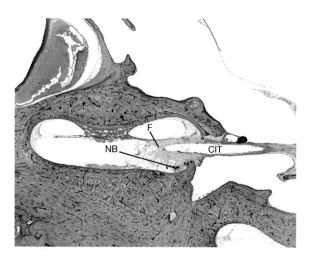

Fig. 16. Tissue seal at cochleostomy. In this 74-year-old man who had undergone implantation of the right ear 12 years before death, the cochlear implant (CIT) can be seen entering the cochlea near the round window. There is a tissue seal at the cochleostomy including both fibrous tissue (F) and new bone (NB).

However, in a study of 21 specimens from patients who in life had undergone cochlear implantation using a variety of devices, there was a robust tissue response in the form of fibrous and bony tissue in all cases (fig. 16) [48]. A recognizable open communication or potential communication between the middle ear and the inner ear was not identified in this series. In addition, an inflammatory cellular response in the form of mononuclear leukocytes, histiocytes, and foreign body giant cells were present in 12 of the 21 cases (57%) and was most intense near the cochleostomy site (fig. 17). It is therefore possible that delayed meningitis after implantation may be caused by a mechanism other than open communication between the middle and inner ears, namely a delayed hematogenous contamination and colonization of the implant similar to the hypothetical mechanism of late infection of cerebrospinal shunt catheters [49, 50].

Histopathology of Vestibular Labyrinth after Cochlear Implantation
The incidence of postoperative dizziness and/or vertigo following cochlear implantation has been reported in the range of 4 [51] to 75% [52] of patients. The vertigo may be immediate or in some cases delayed in onset [53]. In some cases, delayed vertigo following implantation may be similar to attacks of Ménière's syndrome. The histopathology of the vestibular labyrinth in patients who in life had undergone cochlear implantation has been reported [54, 55]. Findings include distortion of the saccular membrane, fibrosis, ossification

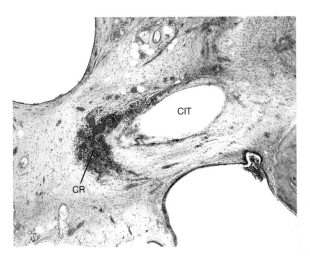

Fig. 17. Inflammatory response to cochlear implant. This 70-year-old man underwent a right cochlear implant 11 years before death. The track of the cochlear implant (CIT) is seen. Close by there is an intense cellular inflammatory response (CR) consisting of mononuclear cells and foreign body giant cells.

within the vestibule, and cochlear hydrops in 59% of implanted bones. In most cases of cochlear hydrops, the saccule was partially or completely collapsed with or without evidence of collapse of the ductus reuniens (fig. 18). There was no quantifiable effect on residual vestibular neuroepithelial cells or neurons of Scarpa's ganglion.

Histopathologic Correlates of Performance of Cochlear Implants

Basic psychophysical and speech-reception measures made in human implantees vary widely in all published series. The underlying determinants of this variance are poorly understood. Intuitively, differences in residual spiral ganglion cell population or function may play an important role in determining the success of implantation. Furthermore, there is evidence for a correlation between psychophysical parameters and residual spiral ganglion cell counts in animals [56, 57]. Ever since one of the early implantees died in 1986 [41], investigators have searched in vain for reliable and consistent relationships between the degree of spiral ganglion cell survival and measures of human performance [for an overview, see 58]. For instance, in a series of 15 patients who underwent multichannel cochlear implantation during life, the spiral ganglion cell counts in the four segments of Rosenthal's canal and the total spiral ganglion cell count were compared with speech reception scores and no significant correlation was found [39]. Relationships found in one study demonstrating that spiral ganglion

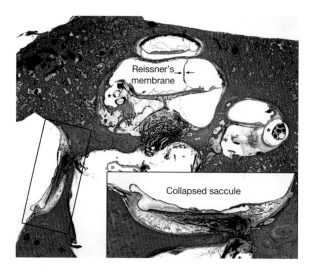

Fig. 18. Cochlear hydrops in a 84-year-old man with a progressive bilateral sensorineural hearing loss who underwent left cochlear implant 10 years prior to death. He had no significant vestibular symptomatology following implantation. There were severe endolymphatic hydrops and collapse of the saccular wall, suggesting dysfunction or obstruction of the ductus reuniens, perhaps secondary to the implantation. Reprinted with permission from Handzel et al. [55].

cell counts account for a significant percentage of the variance in a psychophysical measure have not proven reliable. For instance, in one population the variance in spiral ganglion cell survival does not account for variance in threshold but does account for 60% of the variance in the stimulus level producing maximum comfortable loudness sensation; but in a different population this variance accounts for 18% of the threshold variance but none of the variance in the stimulus amplitude producing maximum comfortable loudness [58].

It is not surprising that the methods used to date have failed to reveal substantial and consistent relationships between spiral ganglion cell survival and behavioral measures of performance because of the known shortcomings of the methods used to date. For instance, the relative sensitivity of a single electrode contact in eliciting a detectable sound sensation will depend on a number of peripheral factors beside the number of surviving spiral ganglion cells such as: (1) the spatial distribution of current elicited by the electrode which will depend on the electrode configuration (monopolar, bipolar, bipolar + 1 . . .), electrode position (basal/apical, modiolar/lateral wall), the amount of new intracochlear bone and other tissue, and the insertion damage to cochlear structures, and (2) the exact position of the remaining nerve fibers in the elicited current distribution. Because complex, three-dimensional factors like these will determine whether a specific fiber elicits a spike in response to a specific stimulus, new methods that are capable of representing the detailed variance in the peripheral anatomy across subjects will be required before reliable and consistent relationships between these peripheral factors and behavioral performance will be established.

Acknowledgement

This study was supported by NIH grant 5 R01 DC000152-25.

References

1   Musiek FE, Lee WW: Neuroanatomical correlates to central deafness. Scand Audiol Suppl 1998;49:18–25.
2   Stach BA, Spretnjak ML, Jerger J: The prevalence of central presbyacusis in a clinical population. J Am Acad Audiol 1990;1:109–115.
3   Hinojosa R, Marion M: Histopathology of profound sensorineural deafness. Ann NY Acad Sci 1983;405:459–484.
4   Nadol JB Jr, Young YS, Glynn RJ: Survival of spiral ganglion cells in profound sensorineural hearing loss: implications for cochlear implantation. Ann Otol Rhinol Laryngol 1989;98:411–416.
5   Penhune VG, Cismaru R, Dorsaint-Pierre R, Petitto LA, Zatorre RJ: The morphometry of auditory cortex in the congenitally deaf measured using MRI. Neuroimage 2003;20:1215–1225.
6   Schuknecht HF, Gacek MR: Cochlear pathology in presbycusis. Ann Otol Rhinol Laryngol 1993;102:1–16.
7   Schuknecht HF: Auditory and cytocochlear correlates of inner ear disorders. Otolaryngol Head Neck Surg 1994;110:530–538.
8   Ohlemiller KK: Age related hearing loss: the status of Schuknecht's typology. Curr Opin Otolaryngol Head Neck Surg 2004;12:439–443.
9   Spicer SS, Gratton MA, Schulte BA: Expression patterns of ion transport enzymes in spiral ligament fibrocytes change in relation to strial atrophy in the aged gerbil cochlea. Hear Res 1997;111: 93–102.
10 Spicer SS, Schulte BA: Spiral ligament pathology in quiet-aged gerbils. Hear Res 2002;172: 172–185.
11 Spector AA, Popel AS, Eatock RA, Brownell WE: Mechanosensitive channels in the lateral wall can enhance the cochlear outer hair cell frequency response. Ann Biomed Eng 2005;33:991–1002.
12 Gantz BJ, Tyler RS, Woodworth G: Preliminary results with the Clarion cochlear implant in postlingually deaf adults. Ann Otol Rhinol Laryngol Suppl 1995;166:268–269.
13 Geers A, Brenner C, Davidson L: Factors associated with development of speech perception skills in children implanted by age five. Ear Hear 2003;24(suppl):24S–35S.
14 Otte J, Schuknecht HF, Kerr AG: Ganglion cell populations in normal and pathological human cochleae: implications for cochlear implantation. Laryngoscope 1978;88:1231–1246.
15 Clopton BM, Spelman FA, Miller JM: Estimates of essential neural elements for stimulation through a cochlear prosthesis. Ann Otol Rhinol Laryngol 1980;89(suppl 660):5–7.
16 Zimmermann CE, Burgess BJ, Nadol JB Jr: Patterns of degeneration in the human cochlear nerve. Hear Res 1995;90:192–201.
17 Bredberg G: Cellular pattern and nerve supply of the human organ of Corti. Acta Otolaryngol 1968;236(suppl):1–135.
18 Johnsson LG, Felix H, Gleeson M, Pollak A: Observations on the pattern of sensorineural degeneration in the human cochlea. Acta Otolaryngol Suppl 1990;470:88–95.

19   Schuknecht HF: Lesions of the organ of Corti. Trans Am Acad Ophthalmol Otolaryngol 1953; 57:366–383.

20   Spoendlin H: Factors inducing retrograde degeneration of the cochlear nerve. Ann Otol Rhinol Laryngol Suppl 1984;112:76–82.

21   Ishi T, Toriyama M: Sudden deafness with severe loss of cochlear neurons. Ann Otol Rhinol Laryngol 1977;86:541–547.

22   Spoendlin H: Optic cochleovestibular degenerations in hereditary ataxias. II. Temporal bone pathology in two cases of Friedreich's ataxia with vestibulo-cochlear disorders. Brain 1974;97: 41–48.

23   Nadol JB Jr: Innervation densities of inner and outer hair cells of the human organ of Corti. Evidence for auditory neural degeneration in a case of Usher's syndrome. ORL J Otorhinolaryngol Relat Spec 1988;50:363–370.

24   Pujol R, Rebillard M, Rebillard G: Primary neural disorders in the deaf white cat cochlea. Acta Otolaryngol 1977;83:59–64.

25   Kerr A, Schuknecht HF: The spiral ganglion in profound deafness. Acta Otolaryngol 1968;65: 586–598.

26   Otte J, Schuknecht HF, Kerr AG: Ganglion cell population in normal and pathological human cochleae; implications for cochlear implantation. Laryngoscope 1978;88:1231–1246.

27   Nadol JB Jr, Xu WZ: Diameter of the cochlear nerve in deaf humans: implications for cochlear implantation. Ann Otol Rhinol Laryngol 1992;101:988–993.

28   Becker TS, Eisenberg LS, Luxford WM, House WF: Labyrinthine ossification secondary to childhood bacterial meningitis: implications for cochlear implant surgery. AJNR Am J Neuroradiol 1984;5:739–741.

29   Balkany T, Gantz B, Nadol JB Jr: Multichannel cochlear implants in partially ossified cochleas. Ann Otol Rhinol Laryngol Suppl 1988;97:3–7.

30   Nadol JB Jr, Hsu WC: Histopathologic correlation of spiral ganglion cell count and new bone formation in the cochlea following meningogenic labyrinthitis and deafness. Ann Otol Rhinol Laryngol 1991;100:712–716.

31   Nadol JB Jr: Patterns of neural degeneration in the human cochlea and auditory nerve: implications for cochlear implantation. Otolaryngol Head Neck Surg 1997;117:220–228.

32   Shinkawa H, Nadol JB Jr: Histopathology of the inner ear in Usher's syndrome as observed by light and electron microscopy. Ann Otol Rhinol Laryngol 1986;95:313–318.

33   van Aarem A, Cremers WR, Benraad-vanRens MJ: Usher syndrome. A temporal bone report. Arch Otolaryngol Head Neck Surg 1995;121:916–921.

34   Wagenaar M, Schuknecht HF, Nadol JB Jr, Benraad-van Rens M, Pieke-Dahl S, Kimberling W, Cremers C: Histologic features of the temporal bone in Usher syndrome type I. Arch Otolaryngol Head Neck Surg 2000;126:1018–1023.

35   Robertson NG, Lu L, Heller S, Merchant SN, Eavey RD, et al: Mutations in a novel cochlear gene cause DFNA9, a human non-syndromic deafness with vestibular dysfunction. Nat Genet 1998;20:299–303.

36   Merchant SN, Linthicum FH, Nadol JB Jr: Histopathology of the inner ear in DFNA9; in Kitamura K, Steel KP (eds): Genetics in Otorhinolaryngology. Adv Otorhinolaryngol, Basel, Karger, 2000, vol 56, pp 212–217.

37   Jensen J: Malformations of the inner ear in deaf children. Acta Radiol Suppl 1969;286:1–97.

38   Nadol JB Jr, Shaio JY, Burgess BJ, Ketten DK, Eddington DK, Gantz BJ, Kos I, Montandon P, Coker NJ, Roland JT, Shallop JK: Histopathology of cochlear implants in humans. Ann Otol Rhinol Laryngol 2001;110:883–891.

39   Khan AM, Hanzel O, Eddington DK, Damian D, Nadol JB Jr: Effect of cochlear implantation on residual spiral ganglion cell count as determined by comparison with the contralateral nonimplanted inner ear in humans. Ann Otol Rhinol Laryngol 2005;114:381–385.

40   Shephard RK, Clark GM, Black RC: Chronic electrical stimulation of the auditory nerve in cats. Acat Otolaryngol Suppl 1983;399:19–31.

41   Clark GM, Shepherd RK, Franz BK, Dowell RC, Tong YC, Blamey PJ, Webb RL, Pyman BC, McNaughtan J, Bloom DM, et al: The histopathology of the human temporal bone and auditory central nervous system following cochlear implantation in a patient. Correlation with psychophysics and speech perception results. Acta Otolaryngol 1988(suppl 448):1–65.

42   Linthicum FH Jr, Fayad J, Otto SR, Galey FR, House WF: Cochlear implant histopathology. Am J Otol 1991;12:245–311.

43   Nadol JB Jr, Ketten DR, Burgess BJ: Otopathology in a case of multichannel cochlear implantation. Laryngoscope1994;104:299–303.

44   Daspit CP: Meningitis as a result of a cochlear implant: case report. Otolaryngol Head Neck Surg 1991;105:115–116.

45   Hoffman RA, Cohen NL: Complications of cochlear implant surgery. Ann Otol Rhinol Laryngol Suppl 1995;166:420–422.

46   Page EL, Eby TL: Meningitis after cochlear implantation in Mondini malformation. Otolaryngol Head Neck Surg 1997;116:104–106.

47   Arnold W, Bredberg G, Gstottner W, Helms J, Hildmann H, Kiratzidis T, Muller J, Ramsden RT, Roland P, Walterspiel JN: Meningitis following cochlear implantation: pathomechanisms, clinical symptoms, conservative and surgical treatments. ORL J Otorhinolaryngol Relat Spec 2002;64: 382–389.

48   Nadol JB Jr, Eddington DK: Histologic evaluation of the tissue seal and biologic response around cochlear implant electrodes in the human. Otol Neurotol 2004;25:257–262.

49   Fan-Havard P, Nahata MC: Treatment and prevention of infections of cerebrospinal fluid shunts. Clin Pharmacol 1987;6:866–880.

50   Ronan A, Hogg GG, Klug GL: Cerebrospinal fluid shunt infections in children. Pediatr Infect Dis J 1995;14:782–786.

51   Buchman CA, Joy J, Hodges A, Telischi FF, Balkany TJ: Vestibular effects of cochlear implantation. Laryngoscope 2004;114:1–22.

52   Steenerson RL, Cronin GW, Gary LB: Vertigo after cochlear implantation. Otol Neurotol 2001;22:842–843.

53   Fina M, Skinner M, Goebel JA, Piccirillo JF, Neely JG, Black O: Vestibular dysfunction after cochlear implantation. Otol Neurotol 2003;24:234–242.

54   Tien HC, Linthicum FJ Jr: Histopathologic changes in the vestibule after cochlear implantation. Otolaryngol Head Neck Surg 2002;127:260–264.

55   Handzel O, Burgess BJ, Nadol JB Jr: Histopathology of the peripheral vestibular system after cochlear implantation in the human. Otol Neurotol 2006;27:57–64.

56   Pfingst BE, Sutton D, Miller JM, Bohne BA: Relation of psychophysical data to histopathology in monkeys with cochlear implants. Acta Otolaryngol 1981;92:1–13.

57   Pfingst BE, Sutton D: Relation of cochlear implant function to histopathology in monkeys. Ann NY Acad Sci 1983;405:224–239.

58   Kahn AM, Whiten DM, Nadol JB, Eddington DK: Histopathology of human cochlear implants: correlation of psychophysical and anatomical measures. Hearing Res 2005;205:83–93.

Joseph B. Nadol Jr, MD
Department of Otolaryngology, Massachusetts Eye and Ear Infirmary
243 Charles St.
Boston, MA 02114 (USA)
Tel. +1 617 573 3652, Fax +1 617 573 3939, E-Mail joseph_nadol@meei.harvard.edu

Møller AR (ed): Cochlear and Brainstem Implants.
Adv Otorhinolaryngol. Basel, Karger, 2006, vol 64, pp 50–65

....

Factors Influencing Spoken Language Outcomes in Children following Early Cochlear Implantation

Ann E. Geers

Department of Otorhinolaryngology, Head and Neck Surgery, University of Texas
Southwestern Medical Center, and The Callier Advanced Hearing Research Center,
University of Texas at Dallas School of Behavioral and Brain Sciences, Dallas,
Tex., USA

Abstract

Development of spoken language is an objective of virtually all English-based educational programs for children who are deaf or hard of hearing. The primary goal of pediatric cochlear implantation is to provide critical speech information to the child's auditory system and brain to maximize the chances of developing spoken language. Cochlear implants have the potential to accomplish for profoundly deaf children what the electronic hearing aid made possible for hard of hearing children more than 50 years ago. Though the cochlear implant does not allow for hearing of the same quality as that experienced by persons without a hearing loss, it nonetheless has revolutionized the experience of spoken language acquisition for deaf children. However, the variability in performance remains quite high, with limited explanation as to the reasons for good and poor outcomes. Evaluating the success of cochlear implantation requires careful consideration of intervening variables, the characteristics of which are changing with advances in technology and clinical practice. Improvement in speech coding strategies, implantation at younger ages and in children with greater preimplant residual hearing, and rehabilitation focused on speech and auditory skill development are leading to a larger proportion of children approaching spoken language levels of hearing age-mates.

Historical Perspective

It is apparent that spoken language development occurs spontaneously in the presence of normal hearing from birth, given a typical linguistic and social environment, and is diminished by the early deprivation of auditory stimulation that occurs with prelingual hearing loss. Before hearing aids were widely available, deaf children missed many of the speech sounds that occurred in everyday life, and teaching them to use and understand spoken language relied largely on visual, kinesthetic and tactile cues. The advent of the wearable electronic hearing aid more than 50 years ago had a dramatic effect on the spoken language development of these children. Teachers soon realized that more normal speech development could be encouraged in deaf children by maximizing use of their limited residual hearing [1, 2]. This auditory approach, combined with an emphasis on early intervention, formed the basis for auditory-oral education of deaf children, as we know it today. New developments in hearing aids and ear molds permitted even severely hard of hearing children to detect most speech sounds, including the low intensity, high frequency sounds of speech, such as the /s/ and /t/. When hearing aids were fitted early in life, and accompanied by appropriate intervention, many hard of hearing children were able to learn to understand and produce speech through everyday involvement in spoken language communication.

Electronic hearing aids were less successful in ensuring spoken language development in profoundly deaf children. Many years of intensive formal instruction by highly trained teachers was often required for deaf children to develop the ability to make use of other sensory modalities to understand and produce speech. Their language development proceeded at about half the rate of hearing children [3], and they demonstrated average language delays of 4–5 years by the time they entered high school [4]. The reported speech intelligibility of children with profound deafness was quite variable, averaging as low as 19% in some studies [5] and as high as 76% in others [6].

The slow speech and language progress in profoundly deaf children achieved with oral methods promoted the development of various systems for providing visual support to spoken English. During the 1970s, different forms of signed English were widely used in classrooms across the country [7]. The 'total communication' (TC) approach reduced the emphasis on audition and speech training compared to auditory-oral methods and increased visual language input, but the levels of English language competence exhibited by deaf children did not improve [8, 9]. Cued speech, a system developed to visually convey spoken language at the phonemic level using hand shapes and placements to complement and for decreasing ambiguities in lip reading, has been adapted to more than 40 languages. This system has been most widely used and evaluated in the French language [10] but has had limited application in educational programs in the US.

Another attempt to improve access to spoken English by profoundly deaf children was the advent of wearable multichannel vibrotactile aids in the 1980s. These aids were designed to present temporal and spectral aspects of speech through a body-worn vibrator. These devices were expected to be valuable complements to hearing aids and lip reading for comprehension of speech in the profoundly deaf [11]. However, no improvement in speech or language skills over those achieved with hearing aids alone has been documented, even after several years of intensive training [12].

The first multichannel cochlear implant system was introduced in the US in 1984 and gained Food and Drug Administration (FDA) approval in 1990 for children aged 2 years and older. Since then, thousands of deaf children have been given access to the sounds of spoken language via a device that is quite different from anything previously available. Both hearing aids and cochlear implants are designed to provide discrimination of speech in hard of hearing and deaf children, but they do so in fundamentally different ways. A hearing aid amplifies speech and acoustically delivers it to the ear, while the cochlear implant converts speech into an electrical signal that is used to stimulate the auditory nerve directly through electrodes implanted in the cochlea. This new technology has the potential to accomplish for profoundly deaf children what the hearing aid made possible for hard of hearing children more than 50 years ago. Now, even children who obtain minimal benefit from amplified speech are able to access speech information electronically through a cochlear implant. The primary goal of pediatric cochlear implantation is to provide critical speech information to the child's auditory system and brain to promote the development of spoken language.

Assessing Outcomes of Cochlear Implantation in Children

The most well documented effect of cochlear implantation is a marked increase in children's ability to comprehend speech [13, 14]. In addition, the use of cochlear implants has provided significantly faster acquisition of speech production skills [15] and language development [16] than the use of hearing aids or vibrotactile aids. Though the cochlear implant does not allow for hearing of the same quality as that experienced by persons with normal hearing, it nonetheless has revolutionized the spoken language acquisition for deaf children. However, the variability in performance remains quite high, and the reasons for that are mostly unknown. Much of the recent research in pediatric cochlear implantation is concerned not only with documenting language achievements in this population, but also with determining what factors might influence the outcome. Documented reasons for poor performance include late age of implantation, poor nerve survival, inadequate fitting, insufficient cognitive skills, educational and social environments emphasizing manual communication and limited parental support [17]. These factors are similar to those that contribute to poor performance in children who use hearing aids [9].

Most parents who choose a cochlear implant for their child report that the primary reason is to allow them to develop spoken language [18]. The use of sensory aids such as cochlear implants and hearing aids is, however, only one of many factors that influence a deaf child's spoken language progress and that must be taken into account when assessing the benefits of cochlear implants. When evaluating the success of cochlear implantation with prelingually deaf children, the contributions from many intervening factors, several of which have undergone change since cochlear implants were first available, must be considered.

Factors Affecting Spoken Language Outcomes

Identifying factors influencing speech and language outcomes in prelingually deaf children is complicated by the fact that both technology and clinical practices are evolving, so that research reports to date regarding the levels achieved by children with cochlear implants may already be obsolete. Furthermore, because prelingual profound hearing loss is a relatively rare occurrence, and because children receiving cochlear implants are even rarer, accumulating a sufficient number of participants to produce research findings that can be generalized to typical implant users is difficult. Large-sample studies typically assemble data collected over a number of years on patients who received implants over a wide time frame. This practice may lead to combining outcomes data from different generations of technology and intervention practices. The following sections describe factors that combine to make spoken language outcome a moving target for researchers seeking to identify the benefits of cochlear implantation for young children's development.

Changes in Cochlear Implant Technology
The technology of cochlear implants has been continuously improving since the Nucleus 22 device from Cochlear Corporation was introduced in 1984 [Loizou, this vol, pp 109–143]. The number of children achieving open set speech perception has increased with implementation of each new technology [19], and their ability to perceive speech in noise has also improved [20]. Speech discrimination, speech production and language scores have been positively affected in children who receive updated speech processors [21] and electrode arrays [22, 23]. The full impact of cochlear implants on speech and language development may be evident only in children who have continuous use of the newest generations of implant technology.

Age of Intervention

Over the same time period that technology has been improving, the age at identification of hearing loss in infants has been reduced from an average of about 24 months to less than 6 months because of mandatory newborn hearing screening now adopted by most states of the US [24]. Methods of determining the degree and type of hearing loss in infants have improved, as has identifying the etiology of hearing loss, fitting of hearing aids and implementation of early family-oriented intervention [25]. Earlier diagnosis and improved early intervention facilitate development of spoken language with or without cochlear implantation [26].

Selection Criteria for Candidates for Cochlear Implants

Earlier, cochlear implants were only given to deaf children 2 years and older with no open set word recognition with hearing aids. Later, the FDA approved implantation of cochlear implants in infants as young as 12 months of age and in children 2 years or older with severe hearing loss. This means that children with unaided thresholds of 70 dB HL or greater and open set speech perception scores up to 30% correct are now candidates for cochlear implantation. Children [27–29] and adults [30] with better preimplant hearing achieve better speech recognition with a cochlear implant. The reason may be that individuals with more residual hearing have more intact auditory structures available for electrical stimulation. Aided hearing before cochlear implantation is likely to maintain the ability of the central auditory pathway to process speech information [Kral and Tillein, this vol, pp 89–108]. Very early use of hearing aids in children with residual hearing may be beneficial because it provides input to the auditory nervous system and acts as a bridge to provide auditory access to language until the child receives an implant.

The average age of cochlear implantation in children has decreased steadily because of earlier diagnosis and changes in selection criteria [31]. Receiving an implant at a younger age has a documented advantage for language development [32]. The critical age dividing better and poorer postimplant outcomes has changed with a decrease in the average age of implantation and has been variously reported [Sharma and Dorman, this vol, pp 66–88; Kral and Tillein, this vol, pp 89–108]. The critical age below which use of a cochlear implant results in no further benefit has yet to be determined, but preliminary data suggest that this may occur at about 12 months of age [33].

Measuring the effects of earlier age at implantation is complicated by the fact that children with more preimplant residual hearing are typically implanted at somewhat older ages in the USA. This is due partly to the FDA guidelines that set stricter standards for implant candidacy between 12 and 24 months of age and partly because of the difficulty of conducting valid hearing aid trials in infancy. As a result, cochlear implantation in children with greater residual hearing is frequently postponed until evidence is compelling that hearing aids will not be sufficient for optimum spoken language progress. This practice may mask the true benefits of earlier implantation, since children implanted at the youngest ages are more likely to exhibit bilateral profound deafness and may be predisposed to slower development of speech perception skills both prior to and following cochlear implantation than children with more residual hearing.

Changes in Hearing Aid Technology

Because hearing aids are noninvasive and relatively inexpensive compared with a cochlear implant, the choice of a cochlear implant over a hearing aid requires justification. Audiologists and surgeons must advise parents regarding the benefit of a cochlear implant over an appropriately fitted conventional high-power hearing aid. In studies using early versions of cochlear implant technology, children with pure tone average (PTA) thresholds of 100 dB HL or greater have been shown to exhibit better speech discrimination with cochlear implants than with hearing aids, but no difference was found for children with PTA thresholds between 90–100 dB HL [14, 34, 35]. Superior performance of pediatric implant users with profound losses compared to children who used analog, linear amplification caused a change in the selection criteria to include children with more residual hearing [36]. However, the question of what levels of residual hearing will result in better performance with a hearing aid or a cochlear implant must be regularly revisited as new developments in technology improve speech perception with both devices. Speech perception assessment of profoundly deaf children that is typically conducted in quiet at a relatively loud level (70 dB SPL) must be adapted to reflect the steadily changing capabilities of newer implants and hearing aids.

Advances in cochlear implant speech coding strategies have occurred at the same time that newer and better hearing aids with digital signal processing (DSP) circuitry and wide dynamic range compression have evolved. DSP hearing aids can improve word recognition scores, particularly for speech presented at low sound levels [37]. Similarly, cochlear implant advances including use of higher sensitivity control settings for microphone input gain [38] and use of higher minimum stimulation levels [39] have resulted in improved perception of soft speech as well [37, 40]. Perception of soft speech may be critical for situations in which the child is not close to the talker. These situations are common in the typical language-learning environments of infants and young children, and it is important to compare the most recent generation of each sensory aid under these less than optimal listening conditions. A recent study that compared speech perception skills achieved by children who use the most up-to-date technologies [41] concluded that digital hearing aids and cochlear implants provide similar access to speech presented at conversational levels (~60 dB SPL) or louder (70 dB SPL or higher). However, the implant offered an advantage for soft speech (e.g. 50 dB SPL) that increased as the severity of the loss and gain requirements increased. Assuming the importance of soft speech for incidental language learning, self-monitoring of speech, and ease of communication in a variety of 'real world' listening conditions, these results indicate that if a child is not making expected progress in developing spoken language with an optimally fit DSP hearing aid with wide dynamic range compression and the unaided PTA is greater than 92 dB HL, a cochlear implant may provide significantly more benefit than a hearing aid. Studies with children who have continuously used the most up-to-date cochlear implant or hearing aid technology from a young age are needed to confirm the impact of improved perception of soft speech and speech in noise on spoken language development.

Child, Family and Educational Characteristics Affecting Spoken Language Outcomes

Characteristics of prelingually deaf children, their families and their educational settings may affect the rate of acquisition of spoken language following cochlear implantation. The impact of these factors on outcome scores may be controlled in research designs either by sample selection or by statistical techniques after data have been collected [42].

Gender
Girls exhibit a verbal advantage over boys in both hearing [43] and hearing-impaired [44] populations. This advantage was apparent in children with 4–6 years of cochlear implant use, where girls scored significantly higher than boys in measures of speech production, English language competence and reading skills [45].

Age at Onset/Duration of Deafness
While onset of deafness after birth is generally considered an advantage over congenital deafness for auditory development [46], when only those children with age at onset under 3 years of age are considered (i.e. prelingually deaf), the advantage of later onset was no longer apparent in speech perception outcomes [47, 48]. It was reported [49] that 80% of children who became deaf between birth and 36 months of age and received a cochlear implant within a year of onset of deafness achieved both speech and language skills within expected levels for hearing age-mates when they were 8 or 9 years old. Only 36% of children with similar age at onset of deafness but implanted after being

deaf for 2–3 years achieved similar speech and language skills. In a group of congenitally deaf children, 43% of the children implanted at 2 years of age achieved both speech intelligibility and language skills commensurate with their hearing age-mates by early elementary school age compared to only 16% of those implanted at the age of 4 years. These studies show that children who have a shorter duration of unaided deafness, whether congenital or acquired, have the best chances to achieve results that fall within the range of hearing age-mates, for both speech and language levels.

Etiology

With a few exceptions, the cause of deafness has not been found to predict postimplant outcomes in children [45, 50]. Naturally, individuals in whom deafness is caused by auditory nerve pathology will not benefit from cochlear implants [Colletti, this vol, pp 167–185; Møller, this vol, pp 206–223]. These are few, and for the majority of congenitally deaf children the site of the problem is the cochlea although the exact cause is unknown but presumed to be genetic in origin. The most common cause of congenitally inherited sensorineural hearing loss in the Midwestern United States is mutations in GJB2 (gap junction protein β2), the gene that encodes for the gap junction protein Connexin 26. The predicted prevalence of GJB2-related SNHL is 22.7 per 100,000 births [51]. A recent study [52] conducted Connexin 26 evaluations of 55 cochlear implants users and related their genetic status to their cognitive, language and reading outcomes. The 22 children who tested positive for Connexin 26 achieved significantly higher scores in reading comprehension and on a standardized block design task (a nonverbal cognitive measure) than those children who were Connexin 26 negative. These results suggest that the isolated insult to the cochlea created by Connexin 26 mutations allows for preservation of the auditory nerve in the cochlea and perhaps central cognitive function, which may explain the better outcome in children with Connexin 26-related hearing loss.

Family Environment

Family factors associated with spoken language progress in children with hearing loss include higher parent education and income [45, 53], parental involvement in linguistic development [54, 55], smaller family size [45], and intact family structure [56]. The impact of these family factors may interact with educational factors, since children enrolled in oral-aural preschools tend to exhibit a more favorable family environment profile [57].

Learning Ability

Children with motor and/or cognitive delays, including mental retardation, autism and cerebral palsy, are slower in their development of speech perception and language skills following cochlear implantation [50, 58, 59]; even children without a diagnosed additional disability exhibit a significant relation between nonverbal cognitive ability (i.e. Performance IQ) and postimplant outcomes [45].

Auditory Processing Abilities

Early development of auditory processing skills, including those associated with attention, learning and memory, may affect the spoken language outcomes achieved with a cochlear implant. The contribution of auditory processing and verbal working memory to linguistic achievements, such as vocabulary acquisition, has already been documented for hearing children [60, 61] and for deaf children before the advent of cochlear implants [62]. It has been demonstrated that auditory memory, verbal rehearsal and serial scanning abilities are also important predictors of speech and language skills in children with cochlear implants [63]. Performance of cochlear implant users has been compared with hearing age-mates on serial recall [64], working memory [65] and nonword repetition tasks [66]. Typically, children with cochlear implants did not perform as well on these tasks as their hearing age-mates, either due to the lasting effects of early auditory deprivation or to the incomplete auditory signal provided by the implant. Correlations of scores on these cognitive measures with indices of speaking rate indicated that slower processing speeds might play a role in creating shorter memory spans. Nevertheless, some children with implants scored within or close to the average range for hearing children on tests of memory and processing speed, and these children exhibited the best speech and language outcomes [67] and were more likely to be enrolled in oral communication (OC) programs after implantation. This suggests that the auditory exposure that children receive after implantation can influence their auditory processing skills and thereby facilitate spoken language learning.

Mainstreaming in Education

Most children with severe hearing loss receive early special education, beginning with individual family-oriented sessions and often continuing into preschool and elementary school classrooms. There is evidence to suggest that access to auditory information via a cochlear implant, especially if acquired at an early age, may decrease the time required for special education and thus result in an earlier entry into a mainstream education setting with hearing children [68]. The proportion of children enrolled in mainstream classes has been shown to increase with each year of cochlear implant use [69]. Earlier educational mainstreaming following cochlear implantation is associated with higher speech intelligibility [70] and better reading scores [71]. These data belie the importance of early special intervention that may serve to prepare children for mainstreaming at a young age. With early cochlear implantation and special educational intervention by 2 years of age, many young deaf children are ready for mainstream school placement earlier, exhibiting speech and language skills that approach those of hearing age-mates by 5 or 6 years of age [72]. Early educational mainstreaming may, in fact, be a result rather than a cause of good speech and reading skills in elementary school.

Communication Mode

Whether children are enrolled in special education or mainstream classes, the communication mode used may influence postimplant spoken language outcomes. This variable is most often dichotomized into OC approaches and TC approaches. Proponents of the OC approach maintain that dependence on speech and audition for communication is critical for achieving maximum auditory benefit from any sensory aid. Constant use of the auditory system to monitor speech production and to comprehend spoken language provides the concentrated practice needed for optimum benefit from a cochlear implant. There is considerable evidence that children enrolled in OC programs have better speech perception, better speech production and their overall language improvement after implantation is better than those in TC programs [73–75]. This is why cochlear implants were first recommended for children enrolled in OC settings, but there has been a trend toward greater acceptance of cochlear implants by families and educators who use TC [76]. Proponents of the TC approach maintain that the deaf child benefits most when signed English accompanies speech. The use of a sign language facilitates learning language through the use of nonauditory means. The child is then able to associate what he/she hears through the implant with signed representations of language supporting development of spoken language. The advantages of cochlear implants over hearing aids for increasing language competence in children enrolled in TC settings have been demonstrated many studies [77–79]. Some studies have documented faster vocabulary improvement following cochlear implantation for children enrolled in TC programs than those enrolled in OC programs, especially when children are implanted young [22, 80].

It is a challenge to determine the benefits of one method over another for postimplant spoken language development because the results may be affected by the chosen sample characteristics. For example, children implanted at younger ages are more likely to use OC exclusively than children implanted somewhat later. Thus, in a study of early implantation effects Holt et al. [33] found that 87.5% of their subjects implanted between 7 and 12 months of age used OC, while only 44.3% of those implanted between 37 and 48 months did so. The selection criteria used for participants in such studies can affect the outcome. Programs emphasizing spoken language may favor the admission of children with certain characteristics (e.g. greater preimplant residual hearing, higher family socioeconomic status, higher IQ) that are also associated with improved spoken language outcomes. Carefully controlled research is needed to determine whether the emphasis on spoken language provided in oral education settings really facilitates speech and language development with an implant, or whether children who make good progress with an implant get placed in oral settings, thus biasing the observed outcome.

A recent study that was statistically controlled for the effects of a variety of child, family and implant characteristics (including all intervening variables described above) examined the effects of various education and rehabilitation models on the deaf child's postimplant development [69]. The 181 children included in this study were 8 or 9 years old, deaf before 3 years of age, implanted by age 5 and had used an implant for 4–7 years. Approximately half of the children came from OC and half from TC classrooms. These children thus did not represent any single program or method, but rather came from the range of educational settings available in North America, and children whose classrooms included greater emphasis on speech and auditory skill development exhibited significantly better speech perception [21], speech production [70, 81] and language [74] skills in early elementary school than children who had received more emphasis on sign language. The extent to which the child's educational program emphasized speech and audition accounted for a significant part of the variance in the outcomes, even after variance due to other education variables, including amount of individual therapy, school setting (public/private), and classroom type (mainstream/special education) was removed. A separate analysis of outcomes for the small number of children who had changed communication mode over the 5-year period following cochlear implantation indicated that children who were successful in acquiring speech in a TC environment tended to move into oral classrooms following cochlear implantation, further inflating the OC/TC difference [75]. Children who depended exclusively on speech for communication had significantly better speech and language outcomes than children who used both speech and sign language.

Overall Language Achievements of Early Implanted Children

The vast and growing literature on the achievements of profoundly deaf children following cochlear implantation indicates a dramatic shift towards spoken language skills that closely approximate those of hearing children. These levels are unprecedented in previous studies of profoundly deaf children who used hearing aids. For example, in a nationwide study of 181 children in early elementary school who had been implanted before 5 years of age, half of the participants exhibited speech that was at least 80% intelligible to naïve listeners [70] and 47% had age-appropriate spoken language skills [74]. Over half (52%) of the children had age-appropriate reading scores [71] and 58% were fully mainstreamed into classes with their hearing age-mates, while another 23% were partially mainstreamed [69]. These results were achieved by a group of children with little or no preimplant residual hearing using early generations of cochlear implant technology (most children initially received Nucleus-22 implants with MSP processors that were later upgraded to SPEAK) [Loizou, this vol, pp 109–143]. The participants in the study had experienced a wide range of educational methods, including both OC and TC approaches and both special education and mainstream settings. None of these children had the benefit of cochlear implantation before 2 years of age. The reported performance levels may underestimate the potential achievements of more recent recipients of modern cochlear implant devices once such children have accumulated comparable implant experience.

Evidence from young children using newer versions of cochlear implant technology show that once they receive cochlear implants, their characteristically slow rate of language development accelerates and they start developing language at a near-normal rate. The developmental gap between deaf and hearing age-mates, which typically increases with age, remains about the same size (measured in units of language age) following cochlear implantation. If this pattern is maintained, congenitally deaf children might exhibit only a negligible delay in language development if they receive an implant early enough in life [82]. Further research is needed to determine whether this normal rate of language acquisition extends to phonetic and phonemic development in speech production, and whether this growth rate continues as the children grow older and acquire complex language, vocabulary and literacy skills.

Many factors influence a child's ability to obtain benefit from a cochlear implant. The amount of benefit is a product of what the child brings to the learning environment, what is provided by the implant itself, and what is provided by the child's rehabilitation program. Our ability to influence intrinsic factors such as the child's intelligence or the family environment is limited. However, we can insure that each child gets the most up-to-date processing strategy with a well-fitted device at the youngest age that is practical, and we can help to provide each child with an emphasis on speech and auditory skill development both at home and in their educational program. Results indicate that attention to all these factors can make a significant difference in the overall benefit children obtain from the use of cochlear implants.

References

1   Erber NP: Auditory Training. Washington, Alexander Graham Bell Association for the Deaf, 1982.
2   Pollack D: An acoupedic program; in Ling D (ed): Early Intervention for Hearing-Impaired Children: Oral Options. San Diego, College Hill Press, 1984, pp 181–253.

3   Boothroyd A, Geers A, Moog J: Practical implications of cochlear implants in children. Ear Hear 1991;12(suppl):81–89.

4   Blamey P, Sarant JZ, Paatsch LE, Barry JG, Wales CP, Wright M: Relationships among speech perception, production, language, hearing loss and age in children with impaired hearing. J Speech Lang Hear Res 2001;44:264–285.

5   Smith C: Residual hearing and speech production in deaf children. J Speech Hear Res 1975;18: 795–811.

6   Monsen RB: Toward measuring how well deaf children speak. J Speech Hear Res 1978;21:197–219.

7   Jordan I, Gustason G, Rosen R: An update on communication trends in programs for the deaf. Am Ann Deaf 1979;125:350–357.

8   Geers A, Schick B: Acquisition of spoken and signed English by hearing-impaired children of hearing-impaired or hearing parents. J Speech Hear Disord 1988;53:136–143.

9   Geers A, Moog J: Speech perception and production skills of students with impaired hearing from oral and total communication education settings. J Speech Hear Res 1992;35:1384–1393.

10   Hage CLJ: The effect of cued speech on the development of spoken language; in Spencer PE, Marschark M (eds): Advances in the Spoken Language Development of Deaf and Hard-of-Hearing Children. Oxford, NY: Oxford University Press, 2006, pp 193–211.

11   Weisenberger JM, Percy ME: Use of the Tactaid II and Tactaid VII with children. Volta Review 1994;96:41–60.

12   Geers A, Moog J: Effectiveness of cochlear implants and tactile aids for deaf children: the sensory aids study at Central Institute for the Deaf. Volta Review 1994;96.

13   Kirk K: Challenges in the clinical investigation of cochlear implant outcomes; in Niparko J, Iler-Kirk K, Mellon N, Robbins A, Tucci D, Wilson B (eds): Cochlear Implants: Principles & Practices. Philadelphia: Lippincott, Williams & Wilkins, 2000, pp 225–265.

14   Geers A, Brenner C: Speech perception results: audition and lipreading enhancement. Volta Review 1994;96:97–108.

15   Tobey E, Geers A, Brenner C: Speech production results: speech feature acquisition. Volta Review 1994;96:109–130.

16   Geers A, Moog J: Spoken language results: vocabulary, syntax and communication. Volta Review 1994;96:131–150.

17   ASHA: Technical Report: Cochlear Implants. Am J Speech Lang Pathol 2003;24(suppl):1–35.

18   Kluwin T, Stewart D: Cochlear implants for younger children: a preliminary description of the parental decision and outcomes. Am Ann Deaf 2000;145:26–32.

19   Osberger M, Robbins A, Todd S, Riley A, Kirk K, Carney AE: Cochlear implants and tactile aids for children with profound hearing impairment; in Bess F, Gravel J, Tharpe A (eds): Amplification for Children with Auditory Deficits. Nashville: Bill Wilkerson Center Press, 1996, pp 283–308.

20   Geers A, Brenner C, Davidson L: Speech perception changes in children switching from M-Peak to SPEAK coding strategy; in Waltzman S, Cohen N (eds): Cochlear Implants. New York: Thieme Publications, 1999, p 211.

21   Geers A, Brenner C, Davidson L: Factors associated with development of speech perception skills in children implanted by age five. Ear Hear 2003;24(suppl):24S–35S.

22   Connor CM, Hieber S, Arts H, Zwolan T: Speech, vocabulary, and the education of children using cochlear implants: oral or total communication? J Speech Lang Hear Res 2000;43:1185–1204.

23   Psarros CE, Plant KL, Lee K, Decker JA, Whitford LA, Cowan RS: Conversion from the SPEAK to the ACE strategy in children using the nucleus 24 cochlear implant system: speech perception and speech production outcomes. Ear Hear 2002;23(suppl):18S–27S.

24   Dazel L, Orlando M, MacDonald M, Berg A, Bradley M, Cacace A: The New York state universal newborn hearing screening demonstration project: ages of hearing loss identification, hearing aid fitting, and enrollment in early intervention. Ear Hear 2000;21:118–128.

25   Ackley RS, Decker TN: Audiological advancement and the acquisition of spoken language in deaf children; in Spencer P, Marschark M (eds): Advances in the Spoken Language Development of Deaf and Hard-of-Hearing Children. Oxford, NY: Oxford University Press, 2006, pp 64–84.

26   Yoshinaga-Itano C, Sedey A, Coulter D, Mehl A: Language of early- and later-identified children with hearing loss. Pediatrics 1998;102:1161–1171.

---

27   Eisenberg LS, Kirk K, Martinez A, Ying E, Miyamoto R: Communication abilities of children with aided residual hearing. Arch Otolaryngol Head Neck Surg 2004;130:563–569.

28   Gantz BJ, Rubinstein JT, Tyler RS, Teagle HF, Cohen NL, Waltzman SB: Long-term results of cochlear implants in children with residual hearing. Ann Otol Rhinol Laryngol 2000;109:33–36.

29   Dolan-Ash S, Hodges AV, Butts SL, Balkany TJ: Borderline pediatric cochlear implant candidates: prepperative and postoperative results. Ann Otol Rhinol Laryngol 2000;109:36–38.

30   Battmer RD, Gupta SP, Allum-Mecklenburg DJ, Lenarz T: Factors influencing cochlear implant perceptual performance in 132 adults. Ann Otol Rhinol Laryngol 1995;166(suppl):185–187.

31   Luxford WM, Eisenberg LS, Johnson JC, Mahnke EM: Cochlear implantation in infants younger than 12 months. Int Congr Ser 2004;1273:376–379.

32   Tomblin JB, Barker BA, Spencer LJ, Xuyang Z, Gantz BJ: The effect of age at cochlear implantation on expressive language growth in infants and toddlers. J Speech Lang Hear Res 2005;48: 834–852.
      speech perception by children with hearing loss who have cochlear implants. Volta Review 2003; 103:347–370.

33   Holt RF, Svirsky M, Neuburger H, Miyamoto R: Age at implantation and communicative outcome in pediatric cochlear implant users: is younger always better? Int Congr Ser 2004;1273:368–371.

34   Meyer TA, Svirsky MA: Speech perception by children with the Clarion or Nucleus 22 (SPEAK) Cochlear implant or hearing aids. Ann Otol Rhinol Laryngol 2000;109:49–51.

35   Osberger MJ, Robbins AM, Miyamoto RT, Berry SW, Myres WA, Kessler KS: Speech perception abilities of children with cochlear implants, tactile aids, or hearing aids. Am J Otol 1991; 12(suppl):105–115.

36   Staller S, Parkinson A, Arcaroli J, Arndt P: Pediatric outcomes with the Nucleus 24 Contour: North American clinical trial. Ann Otol Rhinol Laryngol 2002;111:56–61.

37   Skinner M, Binzer SM, Potts L, Holden L, Aaron RJ: Hearing rehabilitation for individuals with severe and profound hearing impairment: hearing aids, cochlear implants, and counseling; in Valente M (ed): Strategies for Selecting and Verifying Hearing Aid Fittings. NY: Thieme Publishing, 2002, pp 311–344.

38   James CJ, Skinner M, Martin LF, Holden L, Galvin KL, Holden TA: An investigation of input level range for the Nucleus 24 Cochlear Implant system: speech perception performance, program preference, and loudness comfort ratings. Ear Hear 2003;24:157–174.

39   Skinner M, Holden L, Holden TA, Demorest ME, Fourakis MS: Speech recognition at simulated soft, conversational, and raised-to-loud vocal efforts by adults with implants. J Acoust Soc Am 1997;101:3766–3782.

40   Firszt JB, Holden L, Skinner M, Tobey E, Peterson A, Gaggl W: Recognition of speech presented at soft to loud levels by adult cochlear implant recipients of three cochlear implant systems. Ear Hear 2004;25:375–387.

41   Davidson L: New Developments in Speech Processing: Effects on Speech Perception Abilities in Children with Cochlear Implants and Digital Hearing Aids. Washington University, 2003.

42   Strube MJ: Statistical analysis and interpretation in a study of prelingually deaf children implanted before five years of age. Ear Hear 2003;24(suppl):15S–23S.

43   Fenson L, Pethick S, Renda C, Cox JL, Dale PS, Renznick JS: Short-form versions of the MacArthur communicative development inventories. Appl Psycholinguist 2000;21:95–115.

44   Easterbrooks SR, O'Rourke CM: Gender differences is response to auditory-verbal intervention in children who are deaf or hard-of-hearing. Am Ann Deaf 2001;146:309–319.

45   Moog J, Geers A: Epilogue: major findings, conclusions and implications for deaf education. Ear Hear 2003;24:121S–125S.

46   Fryauf-Bertschy H, Tyler RS, Kelsay DM, Gantz BJ: Performance over time of congenitally deaf and postlingually deafened children using a multichannel cochlear implant. J Speech Hear Res 1992;35:913–920.

47   Miyamoto RT, Osberger MJ, Robbins AM, Myres WA, Kessler K: Prelingually deafened children's performance with the nucleus multichannel cochlear implant. Am J Otol 1993;14:437–445.

48   Tyler R, Parkinson AJ, Fryauf-Bertchy H, Lowder MW, Parkinson WS, Gantz BJ: Speech perception by prelingually deaf children and postlingually deaf adults with cochlear implant. Scand Audiol Suppl 1997;46:65–71.

Spoken Language Outcomes in Children   63

49 Geers A: Speech, language and reading skills after early cochlear implantation. Arch Otolaryngol Head Neck Surg 2004;130:634–638.

50 Pyman BC, Blamey P, Lacy P, Clark G, Dowell RC: The development of speech perception in children using cochlear implants: effects of etiologic factors. Am J Otol 2000;21:57–61.

51 Green GE, Scott DA, McDonald JM, Woodworth GG, Sheffield VC, Smith RJ: Carrier rates in the midwestern United States for GJB2 mutations causing inherited deafness. JAMA 1999;281: 2211–2216.

52 Bauer P, Geers A, Brenner C, Moog J, Smith RJ: The effect of GJB2 Allele Variants on Performance after Cochlear Implantation. Laryngoscope 2003;113:2135–2140.

53 Easterbrooks SR, O'Rourke CM, Todd NW: Child and family factors associated with deaf children's success in auditory-verbal therapy. Am J Otol 2000;21:341–344.

54 Bertram B, Pad D: Importance of auditory-verbal education and parents' participation after cochlear implantation of very young children. Ann Otol Rhinol Laryngol Suppl 1995;166:97–100.

55 Cohen N, Waltzman S: Cochlear implants: an overview and update. Otolaryngol Head Neck Surg 1995;116:146–152.

56 Calderon R, Low S: Early social-emotional, language, and academic development in children with hearing loss. Am Ann Deaf 1998;143:225–234.

57 Musselman C, Wilson AK, Lindsey P: Factors affecting the placement of preschool-aged deaf children. Am Ann Deaf 1989;134:9–13.

58 Isaacson JE, Hasenstab MS, Wohl DL, Williams GH: Learning disability in children with postmeningitic cochlear implants. Arch Otolaryngol Head Neck Surg 1996;122:929–936.

59 Waltzman S, Scalchunes V, Cohen NL: Performance of multiply handicapped children using cochlear implants. Am J Otol 2000;21:329–335.

60 Gathercole SE, Adams A: Phonological working memory in very young children. Dev Psychol 1993;29:770–778.

61 Gathercole SE, Baddeley A: Working Memory and Language. Hillsdale NJ, Lawrence Erlbaum, 1993.

62 Bebko JM, Bell MA, Metcalf-Haggert A, McKinnon E: Language proficiency and the prediction of spontaneous rehearsal in children who are deaf. J Exp Child Psychol 1998;68:51–69.

63 Burkholder R, Pisoni D: Working memory capacity, verbal rehearsal speech, and scanning in deaf children with cochlear implants; in Spencer PE, Marschark M (eds): Advances in the Spoken Language Development of Deaf and Hard-of-Hearing Children. Oxford, NY: Oxford University Press, 2006, pp 328–357.

64 Pisoni D, Cleary M: Measures of working memory span and verbal rehearsal speed in deaf children after cochlear implantation. Ear Hear 2003;24(suppl):106S–120S.

65 Cleary M, Pisoni DB, Kirk KI: Working memory spans as predictors of spoken word recognition and receptive vocabulary in children with cochlear implants. Volta Review 2003;102:259–280.

66 Dillon C, Pisoni D, Cleary M, Carter A: Nonword imitation by children with cochlear implants. Arch Otolaryngol Head Neck Surg 2004;130:587–591.

67 Pisoni D, Geers A: Working memory in deaf children with cochlear implants: correlations between digit span and measures of spoken language processing. Ann Otol Rhinol Laryngol 2000;109: 92–93.

68 Francis HW, Koch ME, Wyatt JR, Niparko JK: Trends in educational placement and cost-benefit considerations in children with cochlear implants. Arch Otolaryngol Head Neck Surg 1999;125: 499–505.

69 Geers A, Brenner C: Background and educational characteristics of prelingually deaf children implanted by five years of age. Ear Hear 2003;24(suppl):2S–14S.

70 Tobey EA, Geers AE, Brenner C, Altuna D, Gabbert G: Factors associated with development of speech production skills in children implanted by age five. Ear Hear 2003;24(suppl):36S–45S.

71 Geers AE: Predictors of reading skill development in children with early cochlear implantation. Ear Hear 2003;24(suppl):59S–68S.

72 Moog JS: Changing expectations for children with cochlear implants. Ann Otol Rhinol Laryngol 2002;111:138–142.

73 Tobey E, Geers A, Douek BM, Perrin J, Skellett R, Brenner C: Factors associated with speech intelligibility in children with cochlear implants. Ann Otol Rhinol Laryngol 2000;109:28–30.

74 Geers AE, Nicholas JG, Sedey AL: Language skills of children with early cochlear implantation. Ear Hear 2003;24(suppl):46S–58S.

75 Geers A: Educational intervention and outcomes of early cochlear implantation. Int Congr Ser 2004;1273:405–408.

76 Osberger MJ, Zimmerman-Phillips S, Koch DB: Cochlear implant candidacy and performance trends in children. Ann Otol Rhinol Laryngol 2002;111:62–65.

77 Miyamoto RT, Svirsky MA, Robbins AM: Enhancement of expressive language in prelingually deaf children with cochlear implants. Acta Otolaryngol 1997;117:154–157.

78 Tomblin B, Spencer L, Flock S, Tyler R, Gantz B: A comparison of language achievement in children with cochlear implants and children using hearing aids. J Speech Lang Hear Res 1999;42:497–511.

79 Tomblin JB, Spencer LJ, Gantz BJ: Language and reading acquisition in children with and without cochlear implants. Adv Otorhinolaryngol 2000;57:300–304.

80 Robbins AM, Bollard PM, Green J: Language development in children implanted with the CLARION cochlear implant. Ann Otol Rhinol Laryngol Suppl 1999;177:113–118.

81 Uchanski RM, Geers AE: Acoustic characteristics of the speech of young cochlear implant users: a comparison with normal-hearing age-mates. Ear Hear 2003;24(suppl):90S–105S.

82 Svirsky M, Teoh S, Neuburger H: Development of language and speech perception in congenitally, profoundly deaf children as a function of age at cochlear implantation. Audiol Neurootol 2004;9:224–233.

Ann E. Geers, PhD
167 Rocky Knob Rd.
Clyde, N.C. 28721 (USA)
E-Mail ageers@earthlink.net

Møller AR (ed): Cochlear and Brainstem Implants.
Adv Otorhinolaryngol. Basel, Karger, 2006, vol 64, pp 66–88

·······················

Central Auditory Development in Children with Cochlear Implants: Clinical Implications

Anu Sharma[a], *Michael F. Dorman*[b]

[a]Callier Center for Communication Disorders, School of Behavioral and Brain
Sciences, The University of Texas at Dallas, Dallas, Tex., [b]Department of Speech and
Hearing Science, Arizona State University, Tempe, Ariz., USA

Abstract

A common finding in developmental neurobiology is that stimulation must be delivered to
a sensory system within a narrow window of time (a sensitive period) during development in
order for that sensory system to develop normally. Experiments with congenitally deaf children
have allowed us to establish the existence and time limits of a sensitive period for the development of central auditory pathways in humans. Using the latency of cortical auditory evoked
potentials (CAEPs) as a measure we have found that central auditory pathways are maximally
plastic for a period of about 3.5 years. If the stimulation is delivered within that period CAEP
latencies reach age-normal values within 3–6 months after stimulation. However, if stimulation
is withheld for more than 7 years, CAEP latencies decrease significantly over a period of
approximately 1 month following the onset of stimulation. They then remain constant or change
very slowly over months or years. The lack of development of the central auditory system in congenitally deaf children implanted after 7 years is correlated with relatively poor development of
speech and language skills [Geers, this vol, pp 50–65]. Animal models suggest that the primary
auditory cortex may be functionally decoupled from higher order auditory cortex due to
restricted development of inter- and intracortical connections in late-implanted children [Kral
and Tillein, this vol, pp 89–108]. Another aspect of plasticity that works against late-implanted
children is the reorganization of higher order cortex by other sensory modalities (e.g. vision).
The hypothesis of decoupling of primary auditory cortex from higher order auditory cortex in
children deprived of sound for a long time may explain the speech perception and oral language
learning difficulties of children who receive an implant after the end of the sensitive period.

In one of developmental neurobiology's classic experiments, David Hubel
and Torsten Wiesel showed, for kittens, that a brief period of visual deprivation

during early infancy can profoundly and irrevocably alter central processes in vision [1]. A vast literature now documents the necessity for early stimulation if central processes in sensory systems are to develop normally. Given these results, infants and children with significant hearing loss are at risk for abnormal development of central auditory pathways. Because normal function of the central pathways is a precondition for normal development of speech and language skills, children with hearing loss are also at risk for abnormal development of these skills. The introduction of cochlear implants (and, more recently, auditory brainstem implants) has made it possible to activate auditory pathways and to avoid the effects of stimulus deprivation on the auditory nervous system.

How long a period of deprivation can be tolerated during infancy before the development of central processes is affected? In kittens, a short period of deprivation following birth can affect the normal development of central processes in audition [Kral and Tillein, this vol, pp 89–108]. It is of considerable interest to know the corresponding period for human infants and children. Infants born deaf and who are fit with a cochlear implant at different ages can be viewed as participants in a naturally occurring deprivation experiment and their development provides a unique window through which we can view the effects of deprivation on the auditory system. We have studied infants fit with cochlear implants for many years. In this paper we review our work, and that of others, which provides (a) a timeline for the deterioration of human central auditory pathways in the absence of stimulation and (b) documentation of the plasticity and development of central pathways once stimulation is initiated by a cochlear implant. The time epochs defined by these studies provide the foundation for a rational discussion of rehabilitation options for children with significant hearing loss.

Cortical Auditory Evoked Potentials as Measures of Central Auditory Development in Children with Cochlear Implants

Auditory evoked potentials can be recorded noninvasively from all levels of the central auditory pathways and can provide objective assessments of the development and functioning of the auditory nervous system in young children. For example, the auditory brainstem response (ABR) reflects activity in the auditory nerve and auditory structures in the brainstem. The middle latency response and cortical auditory evoked potentials (CAEP) reflect functioning of the auditory thalamocortical pathways and the auditory cortex. The P1 component of the CAEP has shown promise as a useful clinical biomarker of central auditory maturation in children with hearing loss and in children fit with a cochlear implant.

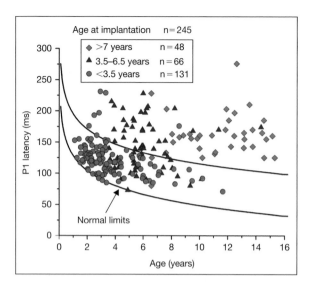

Fig. 1. P1 latencies as a function of chronological age for children with cochlear implants. The solid functions are the 95% confidence limits for normal hearing children [11]. P1 latencies for children implanted before age 3.5 years (early-implanted group) are shown as circles. P1 latencies for children implanted between age 3.5 years and 6.5 years (middle-implanted group) are shown as triangles. P1 latencies for children implanted after age 7 years (late-implanted group) are shown as diamonds.

In our studies, P1 is elicited using a speech stimulus /ba/ (clicks and tonal stimuli are also effective). P1 is an easily identified, robust positivity at a latency of 100–300 ms in young children. P1 is generated by auditory thalamic and cortical sources [2–4]. Ponton and Eggermont [5] suggest that the surface positivity of the P1 response is consistent with 'a relatively deep sink ([in cortical] layers IV and lower III) and a superficial current return'. The latency of P1 reflects the accumulated sum of delays in synaptic transmission in the ascending auditory pathways including delays in the cerebral cortex [6].

Changes in the latency of P1 occur throughout infancy and childhood [7–12]. In normal-hearing newborns the mean P1 latency is approximately 300 ms. Over the first 2–3 years of life there is a large decrease in latency (to approximately 125 ms at age 3) and then a smaller decrease into the second decade of life. The mean P1 latency in normal hearing adults (ages 22–25 years) is approximately 60 ms. Ninety-five percent confidence intervals for normal development of P1 latency are described in Sharma et al. [11] and are shown in figure 1. Because P1 latency varies as a function of chronological age, P1 latency can be used to infer the maturational status of auditory pathways in infants and children. Of particular interest are infants and children with significant hearing loss.

Sensitive Periods for the Development of the
Human Central Auditory Pathways

Studies of congenitally deaf children fit with cochlear implants at different times during childhood have allowed us to establish the existence and time limits of a sensitive period for the development of the central auditory pathways in humans. Figure 1 shows the latencies of the P1 peak in the CAEP obtained in 245 congenitally deaf children who received electrical stimulation of the auditory nerve through cochlear implants for at least 6 months. P1 latencies are plotted against the 95% confidence intervals of P1 latencies derived from 190 normal-hearing children. Children who were deprived of sound for a long period, greater than 7 years (fig. 1), showed delayed P1 latencies. These data are in keeping with data from animal models [Kral and Tillein, this vol, pp 89–108] and provide clear evidence of the effects of sensory deprivation on the function of the central auditory pathways in humans. About half of the children who experienced fewer years of deprivation, between 3.5–7 years (fig. 1), had normal P1 latencies and almost all children who experienced fewer than 3.5 years of deprivation (fig. 1) showed normal P1 latencies. These results are consistent with those from previous studies [11, 13, 14] and suggest that central auditory pathways are maximally plastic (in response to auditory stimulation) for a period of about 3.5 years in early childhood. If stimulation is delivered within that period, then latency and the morphology of the P1 reach age-normal values within 3–6 months following the onset of stimulation. However, if stimulation is withheld for more than 7 years, children exhibit delayed and abnormal P1 responses, even after years of implant use, suggesting that plasticity of the auditory pathways in response to auditory stimulation is greatly reduced after this age [11].

PET imaging studies have provided important evidence regarding the age cut-offs for the sensitive period. Studies such as those of Lee and colleagues [15–18] found a cut-off of about 4 years and are in good agreement with the electrophysiologic studies [11] described above.

These PET imaging studies made use of recordings of resting glucose-metabolism rates in the auditory cortices of prelingually deafened children and adults before cochlear implantation and related these rates to speech perception scores after implantation. The degree of glucose metabolism preimplantation was taken to be an indicator of the degree to which cross-modal recruitment of the auditory cortex had occurred. Thus, the auditory cortices should be 'silent' (hypometabolic) because of years of auditory deprivation. However, if the cortices had been recruited by other cortical functions, then the cortices would not be hypometabolic. Lee et al. [16] reported that the degree of hypometabolism before implantation (which was greater for younger subjects) was positively correlated with the speech perception scores after implantation. In general, children who were implanted before age 4 showed the highest degree of hypometabolism in the auditory cortices before implantation and, following implantation, these children had the highest speech perception scores.

The age cut-off (4 years) is consistent with the 3.5 years cut-off for maximal plasticity of the central auditory pathways suggested by Sharma et al. [11]. Lee's data also suggest that following 6.5–7.5 years of deprivation significant cross-modal reorganization occurs in the auditory cortices. This finding is concordant with the Sharma et al. [11] finding of increased P1 latencies following 7 years of auditory deprivation.

Other studies [19, 20] of cochlear implanted children have found similar age cut-offs regarding the sensitive period. Eggermont and Ponton [19] found that the N1 component in the CAEP was absent in cochlear implanted subjects who had been deaf for a period of at least 3 years under the age of 6 years. On the basis of that, Eggermont and Ponton [19] suggested that this period reflects a critical time for cortical maturation and for achieving useful speech perception. Gordon et al. [20] have suggested that the auditory system in children who have experienced longer periods of deprivation (>5 years) have less potential for expression of neural plasticity (as measured by middle latency responses) than in children who have experienced fewer years of deprivation (<5 years).

In general, there are striking similarities between the critical age cut-offs for normal P1 latencies and the age cut-offs for normal development of speech and language skills. Several investigators [21–23] have reported that children implanted under ages 3–4 years show significantly higher speech perception scores and better language skills than children implanted after age 6–7 years. There are similarities between the critical age cut-offs for normal P1 latencies and the age cut-offs for normal development of speech and language skills. Several investigators [21–23] have reported that children implanted under the age of 3–4 years show significantly higher speech perception scores and better language skills than children implanted after 6–7 years. Consistent with these reports, unpublished observations in our laboratory suggest that children who have normal P1 latencies re: age matched, normal-hearing children, show, as a group, better speech perception scores on the multi-syllabic lexical neighborhood test [24] than children with abnormal P1 latencies [25]. However, not all children with normal P1 latencies achieve high scores on tests of speech understanding and not all children with abnormal P1 latencies achieve very poor scores. As Geers [this vol, pp 50–65] reports, many factors influence speech understanding including amount and type of rehabilitation. None-the-less, it is likely that the neural processes that constrain P1 latency have some influence on the complex of auditory functions that underlie speech perception [26–27]. For a review of sensitive periods as they relate to speech perception and language acquisition in children with cochlear implants see Harrison et al. [28].

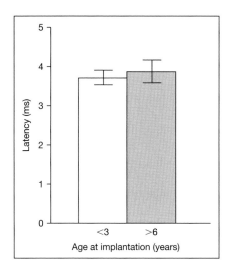

Fig. 2. EABR wave V latency for early-implanted children (<3 years) and late-implanted children (>6 years).

In summary, electrophysiologic and functional brain imaging (PET) data in humans suggest that there is a sensitive period of about 3.5–4.0 years in early development during which the plasticity of the central auditory nervous system is greatest and auditory stimulation delivered during this time is most effective in eliciting expression of neural plasticity. If more than 7 years of deprivation precede the onset of stimulation, then that stimulation is delivered to an already reorganized auditory nervous system.

There is no evidence, so far, from studies of children fit with a cochlear implant that suggest the existence of sensitive periods regarding expression of neural plasticity at the level of the auditory brainstem. Gordon et al. [29] reported rapid development of the ABR response after cochlear implantation regardless of the age at which children were implanted. Data from our laboratory (fig. 2) show no difference in the latency of peak V of the ABR from children who were implanted before the age of 3 years compared with that of children implanted at 6 years or older. Children who were implanted between 2–3 years of age had normal P1 latencies for their age, whereas children who were implanted after 6 years of age had abnormal P1 latencies compared to age-matched normal-hearing children [30]. All the children in this study had at least 1 year of experience with an implant. Critically, even though the P1 latencies were normal for one group and abnormal for the other group, the ABR wave V latencies did not differ between the two groups.

The ABR findings described above (fig. 2) are not consistent with recent data from animal studies that suggest rapid alteration of synaptic terminals in the brainstem nuclei following early deprivation [31, 32]. It may be that measures of latency and morphology of the ABR are not appropriate to assess the

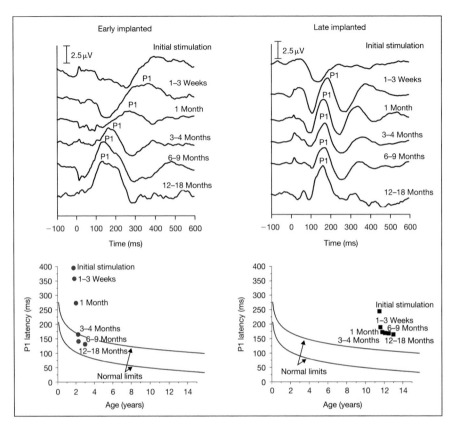

Fig. 3. Grand average waveforms and mean developmental trajectories of P1 latency for early- and late-implanted children. The normal limits are 95% confidence intervals.

effects of deprivation of auditory input at lower levels of the auditory pathway. Another possibility is that lower levels of the human pathway are less sensitive to deprivation than homologous pathways in the congenitally deaf white cat.

Longitudinal Development of the Central Auditory Pathways after Implantation

The brief sensitive period for central auditory development suggests that central auditory development following the onset of electrical stimulation should unfold in a different manner in early- and late-implanted children. This hypothesis is supported by the data shown in figure 3. The morphology of the CAEP and latency change in children implanted before and after the sensitive period are markedly different [20, 33]. At the time of initial stimulation, the CAEP waveform from early- and late-implanted children is dominated by a large early negativity, which is strikingly similar to the long-latency negative potential reported in studies of preterm infants before 25 weeks postconception [34, 35]. This similarity suggests that CAEP morphology and latency obtained at the time of implantation are signs of an unstimulated auditory pathway. Alternately, the early negativity may reflect involvement of nonprimary auditory pathways in the generation of the CAEP when the primary auditory pathways are suppressed [36].

In early-implanted children (fig. 3) there is a large and rapid decrease in P1 latency and significant changes in CAEP morphology in the weeks and months following implantation. Within 6–8 months of implant use, P1 latency and CAEP morphology reach age-normal values (other investigators [19] have presented different interpretations of the rate of development of the P1). The neurophysiologic mechanisms underpinning these rapid changes in P1 latency and morphology are not clear. Animal models suggest that the changes may be related to two factors: overcoming desynchronization between neurons in different cortical layers of the cortex and increasing the activity within the different layers [33, 37].

Examination of the CAEP indicates that the pattern of central auditory development is different in late-implanted children (fig. 3) than in early-implanted children. The early negativity linked to auditory deprivation occurs at a shorter latency in late-implanted children than early-implanted children. Also, P1 latency, when assessed immediately following implant activation, is shorter in late-implanted children than in early-implanted children. Both observations suggest that there is some intrinsic development of the central auditory pathways even in the absence of stimulation.

Late-implanted children commonly show a polyphasic waveform morphology of the CAEP, which may persist for a year following the onset of electrical stimulation. Gradually between the 12th and 18th month after implantation, the morphology of the waveform assumes the unimodal shape of a typical P1 component. However, P1 latencies decrease significantly only over a period of approximately 1 month following the onset of stimulation and then remain constant or change very slowly over months and years. This pattern is in contrast to the rapid change in latency in early-implanted children (compare the bottom panels in fig. 3).

Given the difference in the morphology of the CAEP waveform between the early- and late-implanted children, it is possible that the peak that we describe as the P1 does not have the same generator for the early- and late-implanted groups. We are currently examining this possibility using multi-channel recordings. So far in our studies we have found it useful to label the first, large, positive component P1 as this allows us to quantitatively compare the development of cortical activity for early- and late-implanted children following the onset of electrical stimulation.

Cortical Mechanisms Underlying the Sensitive Period

Congenitally deaf cats can be used as a model system to study cortical activity after the end of the sensitive period. In kittens, the sensitive period for development of central auditory pathways lasts up to 5 months of age [38]. When electrical stimulation is started after 4 months of deafness there is a delay in the activation of supragranular layers of the cortex and a near absence of activity at longer latencies and in infragranular layers (layers V and VI) [39]. The near absence of outward currents in layers IV and III of congenitally deaf cats suggests incomplete development of inhibitory synapses and an abnormal information flow from layer IV to supragranular layers. This abnormal pattern of activity within the auditory cortex is likely to be the basis for the abnormalities in morphology and latency of the recorded CAEP that we have observed in children implanted after the end of the sensitive period. Because the higher order auditory cortex projects back to the primary auditory cortex (A1) mainly to the infragranular layers, the absence of activity in infragranular layers suggests a decoupling of A1 from higher order auditory cortices [Kral and Tillein, this vol, pp 89–108]. Such a decoupling would allow other sensory input to predominate in the higher order auditory cortex in children deprived of sound for a long period. Decoupling of the primary cortex from higher order auditory cortices may aid in the recruitment of the higher order auditory cortex by other modalities (such as vision) [15, 16, 40]. Decoupling between primary and higher-order language cortex in children deprived of sound for a long period may also account for the speech perception and oral language difficulties of children who receive an implant after the end of the sensitive period.

We are currently investigating the functional (behavioral) consequences of a possible decoupling between primary auditory and higher-order cortices. One hypothesis we are exploring is that decoupling would result in abnormal development and integration of audiovisual or other forms of multi-sensory input. A recent study [41] that used the McGurk effect [42] to study audiovisual integration in implanted children found that that the this effect was experienced by children who received an implant by age 30 months but not by later-implanted children. (The McGurk effect is an auditory-visual illusion in which 'seeing' the lips move for 'box', for example, causes a clear 'fox' to be heard as 'box' or a visual /ba/ and auditory /ga/ to be heard as /da/.) The outcome of this study suggests that early-implanted children develop normal multi-sensory (auditory-visual) integration. In contrast, children who receive implants at a later age experience deficits in multi-sensory integration.

The Effect of Prior Hearing Experience on Central Auditory Development after Cochlear Implantation

Age at implantation is not the only variable that influences outcomes after cochlear implantation. As shown in figure 1, there is a 'middle' age range (between 4–7 years), where roughly half the children show normal P1 latencies and the other half show delayed P1 latencies. Critically, there were several children in the latter half of the 4–7 year age range who had age-appropriate latencies. Oh et al. [17] using PET also found variable outcomes in children implanted between ages 4–7 years. This suggests that reorganization of auditory cortices is driven by both the duration of deprivation and another (or other) factor(s).

An obvious candidate for another factor is hearing experience. Studies that have provided evidence for a sensitive period have used primarily congenitally deaf animals and human participants. However, many children who receive cochlear implants have noncongential hearing losses and have 'heard' to different extents before implantation. It is possible that children who had normal hearing prior to becoming deaf from meningitis and children with progressive hearing losses (who initially benefited from amplification) may demonstrate normal central-auditory development even after implantation at a late age. Studies of a population of noncongenitally deafened, cochlear implanted individuals who acquired hearing loss at different times in life provide an opportunity to investigate the extent to which hearing experience prior to cochlear implantation preserves the plasticity of central auditory pathways.

In an unpublished study we analyzed the latency of P1 in 15 children who acquired deafness after meningitis, and who then received cochlear implants at ages ranging from 1.99 to 14.63 years. We found that the majority (7/10) of children, who received their implants under the age of 6 years, had normal P1 latencies and none (0/5) of the children who were implanted after age 6 years had normal P1 latencies. On average, these children had normal hearing for 22.5 months prior to being diagnosed with meningitis. Children were tested after an average of 3.5 years of implant usage. In one case, a child, who had heard for 3 years, showed abnormal P1 latencies after she was implanted at age 7.5 years. These results suggest that a period of normal hearing early in life is not sufficient to preserve the plasticity of central pathways throughout childhood. These results are consistent with studies of speech and language development in children who had normal hearing and who acquired deafness due to meningitis in early childhood [43].

In another unpublished study, we analyzed P1 latencies from 23 children who had a diagnosis of progressive hearing loss prior to implantation. The majority (16/23) of these children showed a normal P1 CAEP, regardless of the age at which they were implanted. On average, these children had pure tone average (PTA) thresholds of 48 dB HL before implantation. In one case, a child who was implanted as late as age 10 years had normal P1 latencies after implantation. It is noteworthy that she had aided thresholds of 28 dB HL for the better part of her childhood. These data suggest that the quality of hearing experience prior to implantation can alter central auditory development after implantation. Stimulation can preserve the plasticity of the central auditory pathways beyond the sensitive period and lead to a good outcome (in terms of speech and language development) even when implantation takes place after age 7 years.

Nonauditory factors that affect success in speech and language development following implantation have been identified. One is increased metabolic activity in the frontoparietal regions that are important for executive and visuospatial functions [16]. Performance on motor development, visual-motor integration and auditory-visual comprehension tasks is also positively correlated with postimplantation speech and language outcomes [44, 45]. On the other hand, increased metabolic activity in the ventral visual pathway, the 'what' pathway, before implantation is correlated with poor outcomes after implantation [16].

Long-Term Development of the Central Auditory
Pathways after Early Implantation

When children are implanted early in childhood, central auditory development (as reflected by the morphology of the CAEP and the latency of P1) becomes age-appropriate within 3–6 months after implantation. It is reasonable to ask whether development continues to be normal over time. In normal-hearing listeners evoked potential latencies and morphologies change during at least the first 20 years of life [7, 9, 46]. We have studied the development of auditory functions for a longer period after implantation using recordings of the CAEP in early-implanted children to find out if the CAEP continues to have normal latencies and normal morphologies throughout their childhood years.

Figure 4 shows changes in the morphology of the CAEP which occur in normal-hearing children during their preschool, school-age and teenage years. From birth to age 3 years, the CAEP waveform (elicited at rates of 1 or 2 stimuli/s) is dominated by the P1 component. At age 3–6 years, a small invagination of the P1 component appears, indicating the emergence of the N1 component. As time passes, the N1 component becomes robust and is reliably detected in

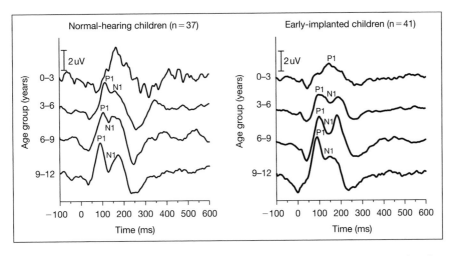

Fig. 4. Grand average waveforms for early- and late-implanted children as a function of chronological age.

the CAEP waveform by age 9 years. As children enter their teenage years and into young adulthood, the relative amplitude of the P1 and N1 components shifts and the N1 component begins to dominate the CAEP waveform. As shown in figure 4 the CAEP in early-implanted children has a normal pattern of age-dependent emergence of the N1 component [12, 19]. We take that as an indication that, in children implanted early in childhood, central auditory pathways continue to develop normally over time.

Central Auditory Development after Bilateral Implantation

Bilateral cochlear implantation is becoming increasingly common in clinical pediatric practice. 'Binaural benefits' include improved performance in noise, binaural summation, binaural squelch, and localization of sound. These benefits are well documented in adults fitted with a cochlear implant, and similar advantages are found in children [47–52]. It is reasonable to speculate that bilateral implantation may ameliorate the effects of auditory deprivation faster and in a more comprehensive manner than unilateral implantation.

As documented earlier in this chapter, we have found that P1 latency and morphology of the CAEP are sensitive indicators of the maturational status of the central auditory pathways. Preliminary data [53] suggest that changes in latency and morphology also offer a window on the benefits of bilateral implantation. After simultaneous, early, bilateral cochlear implantation, the latency of P1 reaches normal limits sooner (within 1–3 months) than after unilateral implantation (3–6 months). Simultaneous stimulation from the two ears appears to create a convergence of the input at the level of the auditory cortex (and lower levels) that promotes normal development of central pathways.

Not all children receive bilateral implants during the same operation. Consider the case of children implanted early who receive sequential implants before the age of 3–4 years. P1 latencies from a second implanted ear are less delayed when that implant is activated than latencies from the first implanted ear. In addition, the latencies reach normal values sooner than the first implanted ear. This is likely conditioned by a starting point for latency that is close to the upper edge of normal latencies.

Children who receive their second implant after the age of 5–7 years (regardless of the age at which they received their first implant) show delayed and abnormal P1 responses even after 2–3 years of experience with the second implant. These data are consistent with speech perception performance in the same children showing that the best speech perception outcome is achieved when the second ear is stimulated by age 3–5 years. Speech perception performance is intermediate when the second implant is introduced between ages 5–7 years, and children who receive their second implant after age 12 year have poor speech perception, despite having excellent speech understanding with their first implant [54]. We infer that even early implantation and long-term implant use in one ear is inadequate to preserve the plasticity of the auditory pathways that serve the opposite ear. Just as with a unilateral implant, there is a sensitive period, or window of opportunity, which exists for children to develop functional bilateral central auditory pathways and acquire effective binaural integration. As our studies with bilaterally implanted children continue, we expect to delineate in further detail the age cut-offs for the sensitive period for bilateral implantation.

P1 as a Biomarker for the Maturational Status of Central Auditory Pathways

Our work has established the existence of a short period in early childhood during which stimulation must be delivered to the auditory system in one way or another in order to achieve normal development of central auditory pathways in infants and children. It follows that hearing aids and cochlear implants should be fitted as early as possible, with dispatch rather than with delay, during infancy or early childhood. It also follows that the children receiving hearing aids or implants will be preverbal. There is therefore a need for an objective

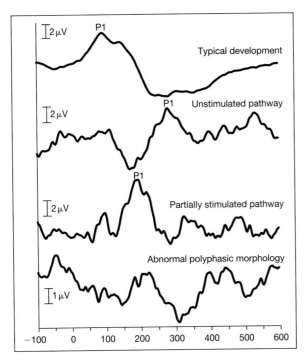

Fig. 5. Examples of P1 waveforms for a hearing child (top), a young child with a congenital, profound hearing loss (second from top), a young child with a mild-moderate hearing loss (third from top), and an older child with a profound hearing loss (bottom).

measure, a biomarker, which can be used to assess whether the hearing aid or cochlear implant provides sufficient stimulation to allow normal development of the function of central auditory pathways. We have found P1 latency and the morphology of the CAEP to fulfill that requirement [33].

Landmarks of Deprivation and Plasticity in the CAEP Waveform

Our longitudinal studies of hearing-impaired children have revealed abnormalities in the CEAP waveform that are reasonably easy to identify. As shown in figure 5, the waveform of the CAEP obtained from young, normal-hearing child is dominated by a large initial positivity (P1). In contrast, initial waveforms following the onset of stimulation (by either a hearing aid or cochlear implant) from children with a severe-to-profound hearing loss are dominated by an initial large negativity. We consider this negativity to be the hallmark of an unstimulated, or little stimulated, central auditory pathway. On the other hand, for children who have a less severe degree of hearing impairment, that is children in whom the auditory pathways have been stimulated to some extent, the waveform is dominated by a P1 response, albeit with a longer latency (fig. 5). In older (>5–7 years of age) deaf children and in the nonimplanted ears of older, unilaterally implanted children, the CAEP waveforms often have a polyphasic morphology (fig. 5). We believe that the polyphasic morphology is characteristic of a central auditory system that has developed abnormally due to deprivation. Finally, there are children from whom we cannot elicit a response because of the severity of their hearing loss.

The morphology of the CAEP described above typically reflects the maturational status of the central pathways prior to intervention. After infants and young hearing-impaired children are appropriately stimulated with either acoustic or electrical stimulation, distinct changes in CAEP waveform morphology and latency occur indicating progress in central auditory development. Over weeks and months following initial stimulation, the latency of the initial negativity in the CAEP decreases and the positive component (i.e. the P1) becomes more clearly identifiable. The latency of the P1 decreases significantly with age, typically reaching normal values within 3–6 months after stimulation (fig. 3). In children who receive a first or second cochlear implant at a late age (>5–7 years), the CAEP waveform often retains its polyphasic nature in the months following initial stimulation. In these children, the P1 may show small changes in latency in the initial months following stimulation. However, very little or no change in latency occurs over the next several years (fig. 3).

Using these distinct and repeatable patterns of the CAEP and the latency of P1, we have studied the development of the central auditory pathways in over 200 hearing-impaired children who were fitted with hearing aids and/or cochlear implants. In the next section, we present four cases to demonstrate the use of the P1 of the CAEP combined with traditional behavioral measures of audiological and speech-language assessment in clinical decision-making.

Case Descriptions

Case 1

The patient was a male child who was born prematurely and perinatally contracted meningitis. He was treated with ototoxic medications and remained in the Neonatal Intensive Care Unit for several weeks. He was diagnosed with a severe to profound bilateral hearing loss at the age 1 month and was fit with hearing aids at 6 months of age. When tested in a sound field, his unaided PTA was 100 dB and his aided PTA was 75 dB. CAEP recordings were obtained at 16 months and 19 months after hearing aid fitting. As seen in figure 6, P1 latencies did not change during this period of hearing aid usage and remained delayed. These results suggest that the auditory stimulation provided by the hearing aid

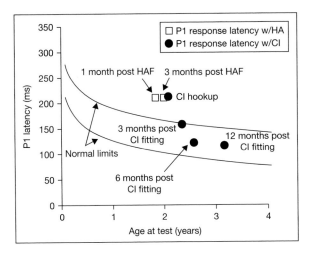

Fig. 6. P1 latency plotted against the 95% confidence intervals (solid lines) for normal development of the P1 response for the patient in case 1. The horizontal scale shows the child's age.

was not sufficient to promote development of the central auditory pathways. The patient met the standard criteria for cochlear implantation and was fitted with a cochlear implant at age 28 months. CAEP recordings were repeated to assess central auditory maturation after implantation. Figure 6 shows P1 latencies at 1 week, 3 months and 24 months after implantation, shown as a function of the child's age. As seen in figure 6, there was a rapid decrease in P1 latency following stimulation with the implant. P1 latency reached normal limits after 3 months of implant use and continued to develop normally when tested 24 months after stimulation. At that time, the patient's speech perception score was 92% using the GASP test. Results of a formal language evaluation conducted at that time indicated progress in acquisition of speech and language.

In this case, the latency of the P1 after 19 months of hearing aid use provided clear evidence that the auditory stimulation provided by the hearing aid was not sufficient for central auditory development. After implantation, the latency of P1 decreased rapidly to within normal limits, indicating that the implant was providing adequate stimulation not provided by the hearing aid. The P1 latency was useful in documenting the lack of adequate stimulation from the hearing aid and the adequate development of the central auditory pathways following electrical stimulation through the cochlear implant. This example illustrates the difference in effectiveness of acoustic and electric stimulation as documented by the rapid decrease in the latency of P1 following the onset of electrical stimulation.

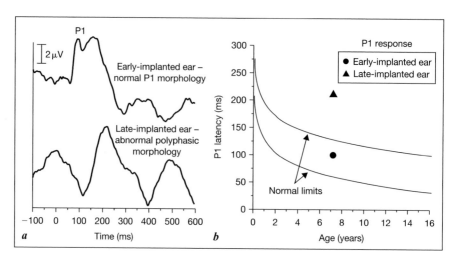

Fig. 7. CAEP waveforms (*a*) and P1 latency (*b*) plotted against 95% confidence intervals for normal development of the P1 response for the patient in case 2.

Case 2

The patient was a female child who was first identified with bilateral severe to profound hearing loss of unknown etiology at 7 months of age. She received a cochlear implant in her right ear at age 1 year 9 months and in her left ear at age 5 years 11 months. She is currently considered a good user with her left implant. When we tested her at age 8 years, her CAEP waveform (in response to right ear stimulation) revealed a P1 response of age-appropriate morphology and latency (fig. 7). Consistent with the normal P1 response, she performed well on the MLNT test of speech perception, obtaining a score of 92%. Implantation of her left ear occurred after the sensitive period. As expected, she had an abnormal response to left ear stimulation with polyphasic CAEP. P1 latency was prolonged even after 2 years of stimulation. Consistent with the abnormal CAEP, she obtained a score of 0% on the MLNT in the left ear.

The CAEP morphology and latency clearly indicated abnormal development of the central auditory pathways that serve the left ear, despite the fact that this child is considered a good user with her right implant. The CAEP findings correctly predicted her poor speech perception performance when using her latter implanted ear.

Case 3

The patient was a male child who was first diagnosed with a hearing loss at age 9 years. At that time, behavioral pure-tone audiometry indicated a mild to moderate sensorineural hearing loss in the left ear and a severe to profound

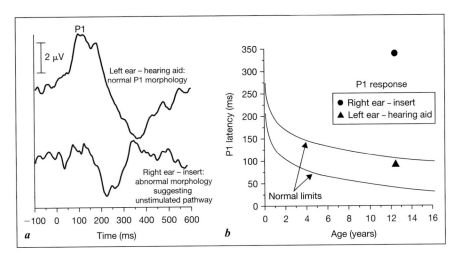

Fig. 8. CAEP waveforms (*a*) and P1 latency (*b*) plotted against 95% confidence intervals for normal development of the latency of P1 for the patient in case 3.

hearing loss in the right ear. Prior to this hearing evaluation, there was no reported history of hearing difficulties. The etiology of the asymmetric hearing loss could not be determined based on the results of genetic testing, imaging or blood tests. In order to determine the best course of intervention, we were asked by the otolarygologist to determine whether the hearing loss was longstanding or sudden. If the hearing loss was sudden, then a cochlear implant would be considered for the worse ear given that the hearing in the better ear might deteriorate in the future. CAEP testing was performed at age 10 years (fig. 8).

Given the mild degree of hearing loss in the left ear, as expected the patient had a CAEP with a robust P1 with normal latency and morphology. Right ear stimulation revealed a CAEP waveform dominated by an initial, large negativity and a delayed P1 component. A CAEP with this morphology is associated with an unstimulated central auditory pathway typically seen in congenitally deaf children. Based on the CAEP, we concluded that the central auditory pathways that serve the right ear did not show age-appropriate development and that the hearing loss in the right ear was likely a long longstanding one. The patient has been fitted with hearing aids and we continue to monitor his progress using behavioral and CAEP testing.

Case 4

The patient was a 3-year-old male child who had significant medical complications as a neonate including RH incompatibility, diagnosis of the CHARGE

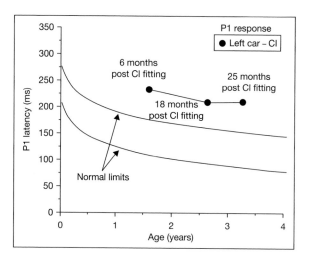

Fig. 9. P1 latency plotted against the 95% confidence intervals (solid lines) for normal development of the P1 response for the patient in case 4.

syndrome, malformed cochleas bilaterally, left facial palsy and swallowing difficulties.

Hearing testing at the age of 1 month using ABR revealed a bilateral, profound, sensorineural hearing loss. Following an unsuccessful hearing aid trial, he was fitted with a cochlear implant at 1.5 years of age. CAEP testing at 6, 18 and 24 months after stimulation with the implant revealed P1 latencies (fig. 9) with only minimal improvement after implantation period and remained prolonged at 24 months after stimulation. The prolonged latency of P1 indicated a lack of normal central auditory pathway development consistent with the finding that the child did not respond to auditory stimuli and did not make progress in oral speech and language development. The child, however, showed progress in acquisition of manual communication. This case demonstrates that not all children implanted within the sensitive period will achieve normal development of the central pathways. For that reason the CAEP provides a useful way to monitor changes in (or lack of) central auditory development of multiply handicapped children who receive cochlear implants. The parents of the patient were considering a second implant. The CAEP results provided an objective analysis of the prognosis, thereby allowing the parents to make an informed choice as they pursued their options.

Our initial clinical results are promising with respect to the use of P1 latency as a measure of central auditory development in children who receive intervention with a hearing aid or a cochlear implant [55]. However, there are factors we need to consider before the measurement of P1 latencies can gain widespread clinical use. These include the effects of audibility, reduced spectral information, frequency response of the hearing aid, and implant mapping parameters on P1 latencies. We are in the process of evaluating these and other factors that may affect the measurement of P1 latencies in the hearing-impaired population. Preliminary results reveal only minimal effects of mapping changes and sensation levels on P1 latency. Finally, we are developing techniques to minimize the occurrence of an electrical artifact generated from the implanted electrode array that appears in the scalp-recorded EEG and interferes with P1 identification [56].

Summary

Studies of congenitally deaf children fitted with cochlear implants, utilizing behavioral tests, recordings of the CAEP and brain imaging, have established the existence and time limits of a sensitive period for the functional development of central auditory pathways. Based on the results of these experiments, the optimal time to implant a young congenitally deaf child is in the first 3.5 years of life when the central auditory pathways are maximally plastic. This is also the time period when introduction of a second implant is most likely to generate a good outcome. If stimulation is withheld for 7 years or longer, the plasticity of the central auditory pathways is greatly reduced. The loss of central auditory plasticity in congenitally deaf children after age 7 years is correlated with relatively poor development of oral speech and language skills [Geers, this vol, pp 50–65]. Animal models suggest that the primary auditory cortex may be functionally decoupled from the higher order auditory cortices, due to restricted development of functional inter- and intracortical connections after the sensitive period [Kral and Tillein, this vol, pp 89–108]. The decoupling may result in recruitment of higher order auditory cortex by other modalities (e.g. vision) as suggested by brain imaging and consistent with the lack of auditory-visual integration seen in later-implanted children. The hypothesis of a decoupling of primary auditory cortex from higher order language centers in children deprived of sound for a long period may explain the speech perception and oral learning difficulties of children who receive an implant after the end of the sensitive period.

Acknowledgements

We would like to thank Phillip Gilley for his assistance with the figures. Kathryn Martin collected the data for many of the experiments. Justin Langran, Rachel Potts and Katrina Agung assisted with various aspects of manuscript preparation.

References

1 Hubel D: Eye, Brain, and Vision. New York, Scientific American Library, 1995, pp 191–219.
2 Erwin RJ, Buchwald JS: Midlatency auditory evoked responses in the human and the cat model. Electroencephalogr Clin Neurophysiol Suppl 1987;40:461–467.
3 McGee T, Kraus N: Auditory development reflected by middle latency response. Ear Hear 1996;17:419–429.
4 Liegeois-Chauvel C, Musolino A, Badier JM, Marquis P, Chauvel P: Evoked potentials recorded from the auditory cortex in man: evaluation and topography of the middle latency components. Electroencephalogr Clin Neurophysiol 1994;92:204–214.
5 Ponton CW, Eggermont J: Of kittens and kids: altered cortical maturation following profound deafness and cochlear implant use. Audiol Neurootol 2001;6:363–380.
6 Eggermont JJ, Ponton CW, Don M, Waring MD, Kwong B: Maturational delays in cortical evoked potentials in cochlear implant users. Acta Otolaryngol 1997;117:161–163.
7 Sharma A, Kraus N, McGee TJ, Nicol TG: Developmental changes in P1 and N1 central auditory responses elicited by consonant-vowel syllables. Electroencephalogr Clin Neurophysiol 1997;104: 540–546.
8 Ceponiene R, Cheour M, Naatanen R: Interstimulus interval and auditory event-related potentials in children: evidence for multiple generators. Electroencephalogr Clin Neurophysiol 1998;108: 345–354.
9 Ponton C, Eggermont JJ, Kwong B, Don M: Maturation of human central auditory system activity: evidence from multi-channel evoked potentials. Clin Neurophysiol 2000;111:220–236.
10 Cunningham J, Nicol T, Zecker S, Kraus N: Speech-evoked neurophysiologic responses in children with learning in problems: development and behavioral correlates of perception. Ear Hear 2000;21:554–568.
11 Sharma A, Donnan M, Spahr A: A sensitive period for the development of the central auditory system in children with cochlear implants: implications for age of implantation. Ear Hear 2002; 23:532–539.
12 Gilley PM, Sharma A, Dorman M, Martin K: Developmental changes in refractoriness of the cortical auditory evoked potential. Clin Neurophysiol 2005;116:648–657.
13 Sharma A, Dorman M, Spahr A, Todd NW: Early cochlear implantation allows normal development of central auditory pathways. Ann Otol Rhinol Laryngol 2002;111:38–41.
14 Sharma A, Donnan M, Spahr A: Rapid development of cortical auditory evoked potentials after early cochlear implantation. Neuroreport 2002;13:1365–1368.
15 Lee DS, Lee JS, Oh SH, Kim SK, Kim JW, Chung JK, Lee MC, Kim CS: Cross-modal plasticity and cochlear implants. Nature 2001;409:149–150.
16 Lee HJ, Kang E, Oh SH, Kang H, Lee DS, Lee MC, Kim CS: Preoperative differences of cerebral metabolism relate to the outcome of cochlear implants in congenitally deaf children. Hear Res 2004;203:2–9.
17 Oh SH, Kim CS, Kang EJ, Lee DS, Lee HJ, Chang SO, Ahn SH, Hwang CH, Park HJ, Koo JW: Speech perception after cochlear implantation over a 4-year time period. Acta Otolaryngol 2003;123:148–153.
18 Kang E, Lee DS, Kang H, Lee JS, Oh SH, Lee MC, Kim CS: Neural changes associated with speech learning in deaf children following cochlear implantation. Neuroimage 2004;22: 1173–1181.
19 Eggermont JJ, Ponton CW: Auditory-evoked potential studies of cortical maturation in normal hearing and implanted children: correlations with changes in structure and speech perception. Acta Otolaryngol 2003;123:249–252.
20 Gordon K, Papsin B, Harrison R: Effects of cochlear implant use on the electrically evoked middle latency response in children. Hear Res 2005;204:78–89.
21 Manrique M: Long term results with cochlear implants in children. Paper presented at the 6th European Symposium on Paediatric Cochlear Implantation, Canary Islands, Spain 2002.
22 Summerfield Q: The Costs, Effectiveness, and Cost-effectiveness of Cochlear Implantation: What have we Learned in the Last Decade? Lecture presented at the 7th International Cochlear Implant Conference, Manchester, England 2002.

23   Kirk K, Miyamoto R, Lento C, Ying E, O'Neill T, Fears B: Effects of age at implantation in young children. Ann Otol Rhinol Laryngol Suppl 2002;189:69–73.

24   Kirk K, Eisenberg L, Martinez A, Hay-McCuthcheon M: Progress Report No. 22, Department of Otolaryngology-Head and Neck Surgery, Indiana University, 1998.

25   Sharma A, Dorman M, Martin K, Gilley P, Spahr A: Relationship between central auditory development and speech perception ability in cochlear implanted children. 9th Symposium on Cochlear Implants in Children. Washington DC, April 2003.

26   Gordon KA, Tanaka S, Papsin BC: Atypical cortical responses underlie poor speech perception in children using cochlear implants. Neuroreport 2005;16:2041–2045.

27   Sharma A, Tobey E, Dorman M, Bharadwaj S, Martin K, Gilley P, Kunkel F: Central auditory maturation and babbling development in infants with cochlear implants. Arch Otolaryngol Head Neck Surg 2004;130:511–516.

28   Harrison RV, Gordon KA, Mount RJ: Is there a critical period for cochlear implantation in congenitally deaf children? Analyses of hearing and speech perception performance after implantation. Dev Psychobiol 2005;46:252–261.

29   Gordon K, Papsin B, Harrison R: Activity-dependent developmental plasticity of the auditory brain stem in children who use cochlear implants. Ear Hear 2003;24:485–500.

30   Spahr A: Auditory Brainstem Response in Cochlear Implanted Children. Unpublished Masters Thesis. Arizona State University, 2001.

31   Ryugo D, Pongstaporn T, Huchton D, Niparko J: Ultrastructural analysis of primary endings in deaf white cats: morphologic alterations in endbulbs of held. J Compl Neurol 1997;385:230–244.

32   Ryugo DK, Kretzmer EA, Niparko JK: Restoration of auditory nerve synapses in cats by cochlear implants. Science 2005;310:1490–1492.

33   Sharma A, Dorman M, Kral A: The influence of a sensitive period on central auditory development in children with unilateral and bilateral cochlear implants. Hear Res 2005;203:134–143.

34   Salamy A, Eggermont JJ, Eldredge L: Neurodevelopment and Auditory Function in Preterm Infants; in Jacobson JT (ed): Principles and Application in Auditory Evoked Potentials. Allyn & Bacon, Needham Heights, 1984, pp 287–312.

35   Weitzman L, Graziani L, Duhamel L: Maturation and topography of the auditory evoked response of the prematurely born infant. Clin Neurophysiol 1967;23:82–83.

36   Møller AR, Rollins PR: The non-classical auditory pathways are involved in hearing in children but not in adults. Neurosci Lett 2002;319:41–44.

37   Kral A, Hartmann R, Tillein J, Held S, Klinke R: Congenital auditory deprivation reduces synaptic activity within the auditory cortex in a layer-specific manner. Cereb Cortex 2000;10:714–726.

38   Kral A, Hartmann R, Tillein J, Heid S, Klinke R: Hearing after congenital deafness: central auditory system plasticity and sensory deprivation. Cereb Cortex 2002;12:797–807.

39   Kral A, Tillein J, Heid S: Postnatal cortical development in congenital auditory deprivation. Cereb Cortex 2005;15:552–562.

40   Bavelier D, Neville HJ: Cross-modal plasticity: where and how? Nat Rev Neurosci 2002;3: 443–452.

41   Schorr EA, Fox NA, Van Wassenhove V, Knudsen EI: Auditory-visual fusion in speech perception in children with cochlear implants. Proc Natl Acad Sci USA 2005;102:18748–18750.

42   McGurk H, MacDonald J: Nature 1976;264:746–748.

43   Osberger MJ, Todd SL, Berry SW, Robbins AM, Miyamoto RT: Effect of age at onset of deafness on children's speech perception abilities with a cochlear implant. Ann Otol Rhinol Laryngol 1991;100:883–888.

44   Bergeson T, Pisoni D, Davis R: Development of audiovisual comprehension skills in prelingually deaf children with cochlear implants. Ear Hear 2005;26:149–164.

45   Horn D, Pisoni D, Sanders M, Miyamoto R: Behavioral assessment of prelingually deaf children before cochlear implantation. Laryngoscope 2005;115:1603–1611.

46   Cunningham J, Nicol T, King C, Zecker S, Kraus N: Effects of noise and cue enhancement on neural responses to speech in auditory midbrain, thalamus and cortex. Hear Res 2002;169:97–111.

47   Muller J, Schon F, Helms J: Speech understanding in quiet and noise in bilateral users of the MED-EL COMBI 40/40+ cochlear implant system. Ear Hear 2002;23:198–206.

48 Nopp P, Schleich P, D'Haese P: Sound localization in bilateral users of MED-EL COMBI 40/40+ cochlear implants. Ear Hear 2004;25:205–214.

49 Schleich P, Nopp P, D'Haese P: Head shadow, squelch, and summation effects in bilateral users of the MED-EL COMBI 40/40+ cochlear implant. Ear Hear 2004;25:197–204.

50 Schon F, Muller J, Helms J: Speech reception thresholds obtained in a symmetrical four-loudspeaker arrangement from bilateral users of MED-EL cochlear implants. Otol Neurotol 2002;23:710–714.

51 Van Hoesel R, Ramsden R, Odriscoll M: Sound-direction identification, interaural time delay discrimination, and speech intelligibility advantages in noise for a bilateral cochlear implant user. Ear Hear 2002;23:137–149.

52 Van Hoesel RJ: Exploring the benefits of bilateral cochlear implants. Audiol Neurootol 2004;9: 234–246.

53 Bauer PW, Sharma A, Martin K, Dorman M: Central Auditory Development in Children with Bilateral Cochlear Implants. Submitted to Laryngoscope 2006.

54 Peters BR: Rational for Bilateral Cochlear Implantation in Children and Adults. White Papers, Cochlear Corporation 2006.

55 Sharma A, Martin K, Roland P, Bauer P, Sweeney M, Gilley P, Dorman M: P1 latency as a biomarker for central auditory development in children with hearing impairment. J Am Acad Audiol 2005;16:564–573.

56 Gilley PM, Sharma A, Dorman M, Finley C, Panch AS, Martin K: Minimization of Cochlear implant Stimulus Artifact in Cortical Auditory Evoked Potentials. Clin Neurophys, in press.

Anu Sharma, PhD
University of Colorado at Boulder
Department of Speech, Language and Hearing Science
2501 Kittredge Loop Road
409 UCB
University of Colorado at Boulder
Boulder, CO 80309-0409 (USA)
Tel. +303 492 1194, E-Mail anu.sharma@utdallas.edu

Møller AR (ed): Cochlear and Brainstem Implants.
Adv Otorhinolaryngol. Basel, Karger, 2006, vol 64, pp 89–108

....

Brain Plasticity under Cochlear Implant Stimulation

Andrej Kral[a,b]*, Jochen Tillein*[a,c,d]

[a]Laboratories of Auditory Neuroscience, Institute of Neurophysiology and
Pathophysiology, University of Hamburg, Hamburg, Germany; [b]School of
Behavioral and Brain Sciences, University of Texas, Dallas, Tex., USA;
[c]MedEl Co., Innsbruck, Austria; [d]Institute of Sensory Physiology, J.W. Goethe
University, Frankfurt, Germany

Abstract

The benefit of cochlear implantation crucially depends on the ability of the brain to
learn to classify neural activity evoked by the cochlear implant. Brain plasticity is a complex
property with massive developmental changes after birth. The present paper reviews the
experimental work on auditory plasticity and focuses on the plasticity required for adaptation
to cochlear implant stimulation. It reviews the data on developmental sensitive periods
in auditory plasticity of hearing, hearing-impaired and deaf, cochlear-implanted, animals.
Based on the analysis of the above findings in animals and comparable data from humans, a
cochlear implantation within the first 2 years of age is recommended.

Electrical stimulation of the auditory nerve by cochlear implants evokes a
pattern of activity which differs from that evoked by acoustical stimulation in the
normal ear. In the normal ear, acoustic stimulation evokes a traveling wave that
progresses from the base of the cochlea to the apex, tilting the cilia of the hair
cells along the cochlea, generating a receptor potential that leads to activation
of the primary fibers through a synapse. This whole sequence involves stochastic processes (e.g. in transmitter release) and nonlinear transformations from the
cochlear amplifier [for review, see 1]. All these processes are bypassed in electrical
stimulation of the cochlea in deaf individuals. The action potentials of the electrically stimulated auditory nerve fibers are strongly synchronized to the stimulus
[for reviews see 2 and the paper by Shepherd and McCreery, this vol, pp 186–205].
The dynamic range of electrical activation of populations of auditory nerve

fibers (defined as the range of stimulus intensities over which the firing rate is modulated) is larger than that of a single nerve fiber because of their differences in thresholds. However, the dynamic range with electrical stimulation is much less than that of the normal activation of auditory nerve fibers through excitation of inner hair cells. This is why it is necessary to compress the auditory signal from the normal range of 40–80 dB of acoustic stimulation to a range of 3–10 dB before it is converted to electrical impulses for stimulation of the auditory nerve. The spread of excitation within the auditory nerve is much larger with electrical stimulation than with normal acoustic stimulation [3]. Last but not least, randomness in the temporal firing pattern with electrical stimulation is much less than it is in the normally activated auditory nerve partially due to the loss of spontaneous activity in 'deaf' auditory nerve fibers [4]. Electrical stimulation at a high rate such as used in modern cochlear implants might induce a slight increase in randomness of the firing patterns because of refractory periods and subthreshold electrical stimulation [5, 6].

Since the activation of the auditory nerve through cochlear implantation is different from the normal sound-elicited discharge pattern, individuals with cochlear implants must learn to interpret this new input.

The ability to use an auditory neuroposthetic device is further challenged if the brain has never learned to process auditory information, as it is the case in congenitally deaf children whose auditory development has not been shaped by hearing experience.

Brain Plasticity and Its Mechanisms

Neural plasticity is the ability of the nervous system to modify its organization and function based on changing external or internal demands. The mechanisms of neural plasticity have been investigated for many decades. As early as at the beginning of the last century, Cajal [7] and later Hebb [8] presented the hypothesis that the coupling between neurons (i.e. the synapse) is responsible for learning by changing its efficacy. In the 1970s, scientists for the first time observed an increase in synaptic efficacy that lasted for a long time (long-term potentiation) [9, 10]. It is assumed that this process is the neural basis for the first steps in the process of brain plasticity.

Plasticity in the Adult Hearing Auditory System

The central auditory system is plastic at several of its hierarchical levels. Changes in properties of cortical cells with training or learning of specific tasks have been presented in studies published during the early 1980s [11, 12]. The

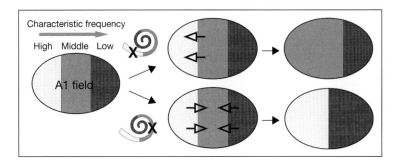

Fig. 1. Effects of restricted cochlear damage on the cortical representations. Damage in the high-frequency region of the cochlea leads to cortical remapping of the middle-frequency representation with the effect of expanded middle frequencies at the level of the cortex. Damage in the middle-frequency region of the cochlea leads to expansion of the high-frequency and low-frequency regions at the level of the auditory cortex.

first report on an 'active' cortical reorganization showed that change (partial deprivation) of the afferent input caused by mechanical destruction of a portion of the cochlea involving a limited frequency range could cause reorganization of the auditory cerebral cortex involving altered frequency representation (injury-induced plasticity) [13]. Frequencies corresponding to the border region between damaged and healthy cochlear tissue became represented in the cortical region previously used for frequencies now in the damaged region of the cochlea – effectively expanding the functional cochlear region into the damaged region (fig. 1). The decrease in the sensitivity of the altered region to the new stimulus indicated that the reorganization was a result of expression of neural plasticity and not acute changes of receptive fields caused by loss of inhibitory drive [14, 15]. The finding of plastic reorganization of cortical tuning curves obtained in studies in guinea pigs was confirmed in other species and in experiments using different methods [e.g. 16–19].

In the auditory system, the nucleus basalis plays an important role in promoting expression of neural plasticity in the auditory cortex. Weinberger and colleagues have shown that perceptual learning in animals involves changes in the threshold curves of cortical neurons (learning-induced plasticity) [16, 20–22], and that similar changes can be evoked by electrical stimulation of the nucleus basalis paired with sensory stimuli [e.g. 23, 24]. Temporal features of cortical units can also be affected by stimulation of the nucleus basalis when paired with sensory stimuli [25].

In a series of experiments, Suga and Ma [26] presented evidence that cortical plasticity plays a central role in inducing expression of neural plasticity in subcortical structures.

As mentioned above, there are two types of expression of neural plasticity, namely learning-induced plasticity and injury-induced plasticity. Learning-induced expression of neural plasticity requires activation of neuromodulatory systems and injury-induced plastic changes are caused by the absence of afferent drive and partial disinhibition of portions of the neural representation maps. The distinction between learning-induced plasticity and injury-induced plasticity, and whether the basal nucleus system has a function in both of them, is currently debated [27–29].

Only limited information regarding the plasticity of higher-order auditory systems is available. Some studies in the cat have indicated that the plasticity in the higher-order auditory cortices is greater than in the primary auditory cortex [30]. Lack of detailed information on the organization of the higher-order auditory fields hampers understanding of the changes that occur in these cortical areas during learning.

Plasticity in the Developing Auditory System

The capacity for reorganization of the brain is more extensive during development than in adult life. Postnatal cortical development involves many processes such as reductions in cell number [31; for review see 32], increases followed by decreases in complexity of dendritic morphology [33], increases followed by decreases in synaptic densities [34–37] and changes in projection patterns [for review, see 38]. Animal studies of the auditory system have shown that partial destruction of the cochlear partition leads to expanded representations of those portions of the cochlea that are functional (especially those neighboring to the destroyed portion of the cochlea). This expansion of response areas is larger in young kittens than in adult cats [39]. Passive listening to a pure tone leads to expansions of the representation of the tone frequency at the level of the auditory cortex in juvenile animals [18], an effect which has not been described for adults.

While newborn babies demonstrate some forms of voice recognition [40, 41; cortical imaging studies: 42, 43, auditory streaming: 44], phonetic specialization to the mother tongue takes place later in life [45, 46]. During the first 8 months of life, the ability to differentiate phonemes from foreign languages is gradually lost (sensitive developmental period for phonetics) [for review, see 47]. Several other sensitive periods exist for language [48]. These processes are especially relevant to the ability to learn to recognize features of speech in prelingually deaf cochlear implant users. The absence of sensory (auditory) experience during sensitive periods leads to a functionally less competent auditory system [e.g. 49; for review, see 50–53]. Similar findings have been presented for the visual system, where it has recently been shown that inter-species face recognition in humans and monkeys is facilitated by passive watching of pictures in early infancy (up to 9 months), an ability that is otherwise lost at approximately 9 months of age [54].

Neural Plasticity with Cochlear Implants

The use of cochlear implants for recognition of speech and other sounds represents a special challenge for the brain and requires expression of neural plasticity to an extent that surpasses the changes that normally occur in an adult hearing person. After cochlear implantation, most of the representations of sounds in the nervous system have to be rebuilt to fit the characteristics of the new coding of auditory input. The outcome of cochlear implantation thus depends on two groups of factors:

Peripheral Factors. The excitation pattern in the auditory nerve depends on the processing of the sounds that occurs in the cochlear implant processor, the electrode type, its position and extent within the cochlea, pattern of degeneration in the auditory nerve, status of myelination of the auditory nerve.

Central Factors. These include the status of the central auditory system ('auditory experienced' in the case of postlingual deafness or 'naïve' in the case of congenital deafness), its plasticity (young subject vs. older subject) and subjective cognitive factors that determine how effectively the subject adapts to the new type of sensory input. These factors determine how quickly a person who has received a cochlear implant will learn to understand speech.

Effect of Hearing Loss on the Auditory Nervous System

In general, input deprivation in the nervous system causes functional and structural changes through expression of neural plasticity [55]. Many studies have shown that hearing loss and deafness cause changes in the auditory nervous system [for recent review, see 56]. The effect depends on the degree of hearing loss (or sound deprivation) and its duration.

Destruction of the inner ear or severance of the auditory nerve in animals has been used in studies of the effect of sound deprivation on the development of the nervous system [57, 58]. If the intervention that deprives the central auditory system of all sensory inputs is performed before hearing onset in animals born with a not yet functional cochlea, it simulates neonatal deafness and results in a naïve auditory system. However, in addition to deprivation of sensory inputs cochlear ablation leads also to denervation effects, and destruction of the auditory nerve fibers may prevent the influences of neurotrophic factors in the cochlear nucleus.

In several laboratories, total deafness was induced by application of oto-toxic substances locally or systemically [59, 60].

Another option to investigate effects of deafness on the central auditory system is to selectively breed species with a high natural occurrence of congenital deafness such as Dalmatians [61] and congenitally deaf cats [62–64]. The advantage of congenitally deaf cats is their similarity to prelingually deaf humans, especially with regards to the slow degeneration of spiral ganglion cells. The disadvantages are the small litters in these animals, and the fact that only 50–75% of the litters of deaf parents are completely deaf.

Morphological Subcortical Changes

Studies in gerbils and mice have shown that cochlear ablation leads to the loss of neurons in the cochlear nucleus if ablation was performed before hearing onset [65, 66], similar to that of activity blockage in the auditory nerve in gerbils [67]. Reduction in cell numbers in the cochlear nucleus has not been reported in any other animal models with hearing loss or in congenitally deaf humans [68; for review, see 56]. Other studies of animal models of deafness have shown physiological and anatomical transneural changes in auditory brainstem nuclei [61, 69, 70]. In cats, chronic stimulation via a cochlear implant reverses the reduction in the response area, provided that the total stimulation time exceeds approximately 700 h [for review, see 56]. Auditory midbrain nuclei of neonatally-deafened animals have fewer synapses and a smaller volume of the inferior colliculus [71, 72]. In the cochlear nucleus of congenitally deaf cats, there are fewer total terminal ramifications, smaller density of synaptic vesicles, and larger presynaptic and postsynaptic areas compared with hearing animals [e.g. 73; for humans, see 74]. These deficits in the cochlear nucleus are at least partially reversible through chronic electrical stimulation of the auditory nerve via a cochlear implant [75].

Functional Subcortical Changes

Pinna orientation reflexes could be elicited by electrical stimulation of the auditory nerve using a cochlear implant in both neonatally deafened and congenitally deaf cats [76–78]. The threshold of electrically evoked brainstem responses is higher in neonatally deafened cats compared with hearing cats [72, 79] while this was not observed in congenitally deaf cats [49]. Temporal jitter of the responses from neurons in the inferior colliculus is increased in neonatally deafened animals [80], and that could contribute to the observed increase in the detectability thresholds of electrically evoked auditory brainstem responses (EABR). The thresholds of the EABR in congenitally deaf cats are not significantly different from those of hearing cats with cochlear implants [49], perhaps because the congenitally deaf cats do not express the extensive degeneration of the spiral ganglion cells found in neonatally deafened cats [72]. Other characteristics of cells in the inferior colliculus, such as the internuclear projection pattern and the nucleotopic projections, were present in congenitally deaf cats [81].

Chronic Cochlear Implantation and Effects on Subcortical Nuclei

Chronic electrical stimulation through a cochlear implant applying a sequence of pulses at a constant repetition rate over several hours per day can affect the properties of subcortical nuclei. For example, the bandwidth of the electrical spatial tuning curves increases significantly after chronic electrical stimulation through a single electrode [79]. Specifically, the representation of the chronically stimulated cochlear region in the inferior colliculus expands and inhibitory responses from neurons in the inferior colliculus increase after chronic electrical stimulation [76]. Therefore, the downregulation of inhibition in the afferent auditory system after auditory deprivation [82, 83] may be counteracted by chronic electrostimulation.

The shortest latency of the responses from neurons in the inferior colliculus decreased slightly but significantly in neonatally deafened cats after chronic stimulation by a cochlear implant, and the onset latency became shorter than in hearing cats in response to stimulation by a cochlear implant [76; for humans, compare 84]. Also, the occurrence of long-latency responses increased in the inferior colliculus of the chronically stimulated group, and that is assumed to be caused by increased descending input from the cerebral cortex. When the stimulation consisted of sequences of pulses presented at a low rate for several hours a day, no change in temporal properties of units in the inferior colliculus was observed. However, when the stimuli were amplitude- and frequency-modulated pulse trains with a frequency of 300 Hz, the temporal response properties in the inferior colliculus changed significantly [85, 86]. The maximum frequency of the stimulation that these neurons could follow increased from approximately 200 to 600 pulses per second, a sign of expression of neural plasticity in the auditory midbrain regarding the temporal properties of responses.

A study that compared the responses from subcortical structures using chronic electrical stimulation in adult deafened cats with those of neonatally deafened animals did not support the theory of a sensitive period for expansion of spatial representation of frequency tuning or changes in thresholds [87].

Chronic Cochlear Implantation and Effects on the Auditory Cortex

The gross morphology of the primary auditory cortex in naïve, unstimulated congenitally deaf cats and neonatally deafened cats appears to be largely preserved over time. However, cells in the primary field (A1), show a slightly (but significantly) increased spontaneous activity compared to those in hearing animals [88]. The primary auditory cortex remains responsive to cochlear implant stimulation of the auditory nerve even in adult, congenitally deaf or neonatally deafened animals [89, 90]. The range of latencies of unit responses is not significantly different between deaf and hearing animals. Latency-intensity functions and rate-intensity functions are similar [89]. A tendency towards steeper amplitude-intensity functions for local field potentials has, however, been observed in congenitally deaf cats [49]. All this may seem surprising because the cortical specificity of some areas in normal-hearing animals is lost after sound deprivation and cross-modal interaction may occur [91].

A rudimentary cochleotopic gradient in the primary auditory cortex is present even in congenitally deaf cats [90]. Similarly, the nucleotopic organization of the projection between the thalamus and the primary auditory cortex is preserved in pharmacologically deafened animals [92], but the rudimentary cochleotopy was considerably smeared in long-term deafened animals [93]. It is unknown if this is caused by auditory nerve degeneration in this particular animal model of deafness.

However, some functional deficits have been identified in the primary auditory cortex of deaf animals. The threshold of cells in the primary auditory cortex is lower in neonatally and congenitally deaf cats than in acutely deafened hearing animals [93, 49], representing a 'hypersensitivity' of the auditory system to auditory inputs. Auditory brainstem responses obtained in the same congenitally deaf cats showed no signs of hypersensitivity, indicating that the physiological abnormalities that caused the hypersensitivity are located at the thalamocortical level [49]. A downregulation of inhibition in the auditory cortex has been noted in congenitally deaf cats causing changes in long-latency (rebound) responses in the auditory cortex [49].

Studies of activity in the specific layers of the primary auditory cortex in congenitally deaf cats stimulated through a cochlear implant [94] revealed that the cortical modules in the primary auditory cortex do not activate synchronously, which is regarded to be essential for proper functioning of the cortical columns [95, 96]. The decreased synaptic activity in the cortex in deaf animals is likely to be caused by the desynchronization of neurons in the cortical columns [94]. The reductions seen in the activity of the infragranular layers which send projections to the thalamus and other subcortical nuclei indicate a decrease in activity in descending projections from the higher auditory cortex [for review, see 97]. This projection is essential for the so-called 'cognitive modulation' of activity in primary auditory cortex, which further controls the relay of activity from the thalamus to the higher-order areas [compare 98]. Further, the thalamocorticothalamic loops play a role in short-term memory in the auditory system, and allow the association of stimuli coming successively into the auditory system, and this function is compromised in congenitally deaf cats.

Processing in the auditory cerebral cortex plays an important role in cognitive functions related to hearing. Biologically meaningful auditory stimuli are expected to cause great changes in the function of the auditory cortex through expression of neural plasticity. In studies of the effect of auditory experience in implanted cats using biologically meaningful stimuli delivered via portable single-channel speech processors, several forms of reorganization of the primary auditory cortex were demonstrated.

The animals were congenitally deaf, and implanted with a single electrode in the cochlea at the age of 2–6 months (as a comparison, hearing cats are born deaf, gain their hearing function around postnatal day 10, and become sexually mature between 4 and 6 months of age). The cochlear implant processors that were used in these experiments were similar to single-channel Vienna-type speech processors (using the compressed analogue coding strategy). All ambient and self-produced sounds above 65 dB SPL within the range of 125–8,000 Hz were coded in the electrical stimulation of the cochleae of these animals. Automatic gain control was used to limit the output to a dynamic range of 10 dB. The processors were fitted to the animals individually within a few days after implantation using the threshold of the pinna orientation reflex to set the gain. The animals were allowed to move freely on a daily basis. The animals were conditioned to respond to a pure tone using food rewards to make them aware of the newly-gained auditory input and to promote the use of audition for control of behavior. The animals learned the auditory task within 3–20 conditioning sessions [77] and they responded to ambient sounds generated during feeding and care. Animals were stimulated for 1–5 months, and after that their auditory cortices were investigated using electrophysiological recordings in acute experiments after which they were sacrificed and their brains prepared for morphologic studies.

The active cortical area expanded substantially and significantly, up to a factor of approximately 5 (sic), in direct proportion with the duration of auditory experience (fig. 2) [50, 77]. The morphology of the local field potentials recorded in the most activated region of the auditory cortex became more similar to that of normal hearing animals, the long-latency responses increased in

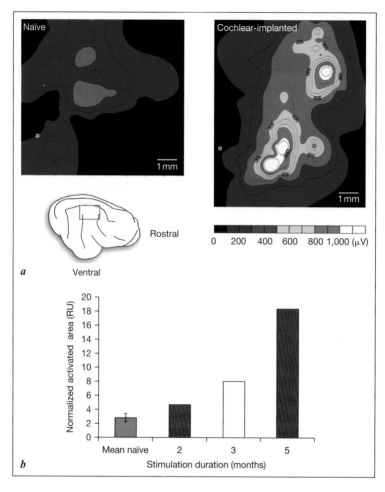

Fig. 2. Expansion of the activated cortical area after chronic electrical stimulation with a cochlear implant. Cortical maps were obtained on anaesthetized animals with monopolar electrical pulsatile stimulation (200 µs/phase, 10 dB over the lowest cortical threshold) and recordings with glass microelectrodes at approximately 150 recording positions within the A1 cortex (inset of the brain with the marked recorded area). ***a*** Data obtained from congenitally deaf cats. Left: naïve animal (not chronically stimulated). Right: Animal implanted at 3 months and stimulated for 5 months. ***b*** Bar chart with the mean normalized cortical activated area in adult naïve congenitally deaf animals (n = 5), a congenitally deaf cat implanted at 3 months and stimulated for 2 months, a neonatally deafened cat implanted at 3 months and stimulated for 3 months, and a congenitally deaf cat implanted at 3 months and stimulated for 5 months. Data show that the results on chronically stimulated animals are consistent between neonatally deafened and congenitally deaf cats, and that the active cortical areas expand with increasing stimulation duration [compare 78]. RU = Relative units.

amplitude. Single- and multi-unit recordings revealed more complex response patterns with variable rate-intensity functions [50], demonstrating that the same unit responded differently to different stimuli, and that the response to the same stimulus differed among the cells from which recordings were made [77]. These results, which were different from those observed in deaf animals, were interpreted to indicate the development of feature detectors in the primary auditory cortex of these chronically-stimulated congenitally deaf cats. The most extensive changes in the gross synaptic activity occurred in the supragranular layers II and III [77], which are known for their high capacity for plastic reorganization [99]. However, the activity in infragranular layers also increased, leading to a normalized pattern of activity within entire cortical columns.

This functional maturation only occurred in the animals that were implanted and chronically stimulated early in life. The later the animals were implanted the smaller were the effects of chronic electrical stimulation on several plasticity measures (i.e. from the age of 2.5 to 6 months after birth, thus adulthood; fig. 3), demonstrating a sensitive developmental period [50, 78]. The older the animals were at the time of implantation, the smaller were the expansions of cortical areas that occurred after chronic electrical stimulation, and the morphology of the field potentials in terms of longer-latency waves matured less completely. Latencies of middle-latency responses did not normalize after chronic electrical stimulation in animals that were implanted late during development or in adulthood.

In summary, most of the signs of plastic reorganization that occurred after cochlear implant stimulation became less pronounced the later in life the stimulation was begun. This is in agreement with many other studies of neurophysiological changes caused by expression of neural plasticity induced during the sensitive period for speech comprehension in prelingually deaf children [100; see also the paper by Sharma and Dorman, this vol, pp 66–88]. As a sensitive period in the midbrain has not yet been found with cochlear implant stimulation [101, 102], it appears likely that this phenomenon is of thalamocortical origin.

The results of the studies discussed above provide information about the optimal age for implantation of prelingually deaf children. Studies have indicated that the developmental sensitive period overlaps with the time during which neural circuits are functionally established, further coinciding with the time where there is a rapid increase in gross synaptic currents [synaptic currents, cat auditory cortex: 49; rapid synaptogenesis, cat visual cortex: 35, 103; synaptogenesis, human visual and auditory cortex: 37] and also with the increase in dendritic branching that occur during normal development [human visual and auditory cortex: 33]. The increase in gross synaptic currents during development is the process most extensively affected by deafness [for study in cats, see 49]. There is also a temporal

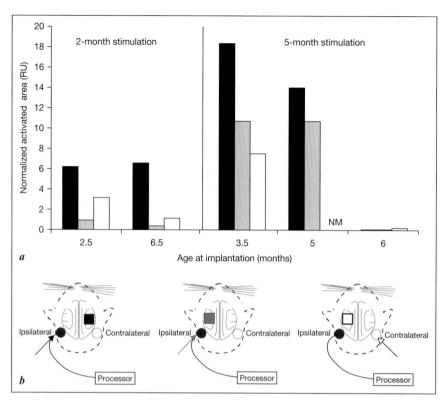

Fig. 3. *a* Effect of increasing age at implantation on the capacity for plastic reorganization. Bars show the activated areas determined at the cortex contralateral to the chronically stimulated ear with stimulation of this ('trained') ear (black), areas determined at the cortex ipsilateral to the 'trained ear' with stimulation of this ear (grey), and areas determined at the cortex ipsilateral to the 'trained ear' with stimulation of the other ('untrained') ear (white). With increasing age at implantation, the activated cortical area decreases, demonstrating a sensitive developmental period. The same effect was shown on latencies of the largest middle-latency wave (Pa) of the field potential. *b* Drawing indicating the stimulation and recording site. Arrows point to the ear that was stimulated to obtain the map, boxes show the position of the cortical recordings. The chronically stimulated ear is marked by the black circle connected to the sound processor. NM = Not measured; RU = relative units. For details, compare Kral et al. [78].

overlap between the time of decrease in synaptic densities that follows and the decrease in gross synaptic currents as shown in experiments in cats [35, 49, 78, 103]. The time course of the normal synaptogenesis in the human auditory cortex is well known: it continues from birth up to 4 years [33, 37]. This phase is the most sensitive to auditory deprivation, at least in functional measures [for study in cats, see 49]. Therefore, and in agreement with electrophysiology in cochlear-implanted children [104–107], it is advisable to perform cochlear implantation before the age of 4 years in the congenitally deaf children. However, since the most rapid increase in synaptogenesis takes place within the first 1–2 years of age, by extrapolation from the cat functional data it may be suggested that the best benefit from cochlear implantation can be expected when implantation of congenitally deaf children is done at 1–2 years of age.

Cross-Modal Reorganization in Deafness

Congenital or perinatal deprivation leaves large portions of the central auditory system without an appropriate sensory stimulus. Do the nuclei of the afferent auditory system, when deprived of adequate inputs, take over new functions? At present, such reorganization in the subcortical lemniscal structures has not been demonstrated. Subcortical cross-modal reorganizations have only been demonstrated after destruction of a part of the normal auditory pathways (e.g. aspiration of inferior colliculus leads to cross-modal reorganization of thalamic inputs) [108–111; for review, see 112]. With such manipulations, natural inputs to other structures are destroyed. This leaves unoccupied synaptic space for inputs from other sensory systems, and axons may be redirected to new, atypical targets.

In this respect, the cortex differs from the subcortical auditory system [113]. While cross-modal interaction does not occur normally in the primary auditory cortex (A1) in adults, it occurs naturally in the secondary cortices that receive input from dorsal thalamus [compare also 114, 115].

In congenitally deaf individuals, visually-presented sign language activates the auditory cortex [116, 117]. A cross-modal reorganization was also demonstrated for nonlanguage (moving) visual stimuli [118], showing that the parts of the cortex devoted to auditory stimuli also process nonlinguistic visual inputs. This is in line with the evidence of superior visual performance of congenitally deaf individuals that has been reported in several studies which have been comprehensively reviewed by Bavelier and Neville [91]. Also, spontaneous glucose metabolism in the higher-order auditory cortical areas in prelingually deaf children increases with age, and is negatively proportional to speech comprehension after cochlear implantation, which has been interpreted as a sign of cross-modal reorganization [119].

The only study, which would indicate partial cross-modal reorganization of the primary auditory cortex, is that of Finney et al. [118]. These authors reported that a 'few voxels' of fMRI images in the right (but none in the left) primary auditory cortex were activated by moving visual stimuli in congenitally deaf adults. All other active voxels were located outside the primary auditory cortex in the higher-order auditory areas [see also 117]. This latter finding corresponds to findings with visual stimulation in hearing humans, where the absence of activation of the primary auditory cortex by visual speech-relevant stimuli has been reported [120]. In neither awake nor anaesthetized congenitally deaf cats could activation be elicited with visual flashes or phase-reversal gratings of different spatial frequencies and orientations [88, 121].

Interestingly, congenitally deaf individuals with cochlear implants and electrical stimulation of the auditory nerve have shown significantly less activation of higher-order cortical areas than postlingually deafened individuals [122, 123]. Based on these data, and the reduction in synaptic activity in infragranular layers of congenitally deaf cats [49, 94], we propose that the primary auditory cortex de-couples functionally from the higher-order auditory cortex as a result of congenital deafness. The higher-order auditory cortex may then undergo cross-modal reorganization.

The results discussed above have relevance for decisions regarding cochlear implants in congenitally deaf children. One question that has often been asked is whether the caretakers of children with cochlear implants should keep signing with these children, or if this would be counterproductive for learning and maintaining a language through spoken words using the cochlear implant? Arguments for both alternatives have been made. Signs accompanying spoken language might facilitate learning by appropriately activating the semantic networks in the brain, thereby facilitating the coupling of the activity in the auditory system with the associative language networks already established in the brain. On the other hand, signing might prevent the reassignment of higher-order auditory cortex to the auditory modality, and thus it may be counterproductive in learning spoken language. The final decision between these alternatives can only be made after further data and clinical evidence have been gathered. Until then, abandoning signing may be considered in order to prevent its possible adverse effects.

Conclusions

Expression of neural plasticity is important for achieving the benefit from cochlear implants. The data presented here and in the paper by Sharma and Dorman [this vol, pp 66–88] demonstrate the extensive ability of the auditory system to process input from cochlear implants. Changes are localized in the afferent auditory system and in the cerebral cortex. The cortical reorganizations may direct the subcortical changes. Since functional development of the auditory nervous system requires auditory experience, congenital (prelingual) deafness results in a functionally incompetent (naïve) auditory cerebral cortex.

Early auditory input is important for restoring the ability of the naïve auditory cortex and subcortical auditory structures to adequately process sensory input. It is important that sensory input is established early in life while synaptic properties are immature and the synaptic densities are high in the cerebral cortex and other sensory structures in the brain because that provides a higher 'range' of possible plastic reorganizations of synaptic transmission and wiring pattern than what is available later in life. In prelingually deaf individuals, higher-order auditory areas can take over new functions, and over time cross-modal reorganization may occur. A sensitive period for recovery from deafness of approximately 4 years of age has been identified and research indicates that it would be advantageous to perform cochlear implantation before the end of the 2nd year of life, but at the latest within the 4th year of life in prelingually deaf individuals. When bilateral implantation is done, the second ear should be implanted before the end of the sensitive period, but simultaneous bilateral implantations appear to be the optimal procedure.

Acknowledgements

Preparation of this paper and some of the research reported were supported by the Deutsche Forschungsgemeinschaft. The authors wish to thank Dr. C. Garnham and Dr. A. R. Moller for critical comments and suggestions on an earlier version of this review.

References

1   Santos-Sacchi J: New tunes from Corti's organ: the outer hair cell boogie rules. Curr Opin Neurobiol 2003;13:459–468.
2   Hartmann R, Klinke R: Response characteristics of nerve fibers to patterned electrical stimulation; in Miller JM, Spelman FA (eds): Cochlear Implants. Models of the Electrically Stimulated Ear. New York, Springer, 1990, pp 135–160.
3   Kral A, Hartmann R, Mortazavi D, Klinke R: Spatial resolution of cochlear implants: the electrical field and excitation of auditory afferents. Hear Res 1998;121:11–28.
4   Hartmann R, Topp G, Klinke R: Discharge patterns of cat primary auditory fibers with electrical stimulation of the cochlea. Hear Res 1984;13:47–62.
5   Rubinstein JT, Miller CA: How do cochlear prostheses work? Curr Opin Neurobiol 1999;9: 399–404.
6   Rubinstein JT, Wilson BS, Finley CC, Abbas PJ: Pseudospontaneous activity: stochastic independence of auditory nerve fibers with electrical stimulation. Hear Res 1999;127:108–118.
7   Cajal SR: Histologie du Systeme Nerveux de l'Homme et de Vertebres. Paris, Malone, 1911.
8   Hebb DO: The Organization of Behavior. New York, Wiley, 1949.
9   Bliss TV, Gardner-Medwin AR: Long-lasting potentiation of synaptic transmission in the dentate area of the unanaestetized rabbit following stimulation of the perforant path. J Physiol 1973;232:357–374.
10 Bliss TV, Lomo T: Long-lasting potentiation of synaptic transmission in the dentate area of the anaesthetized rabbit following stimulation of the perforant path. J Physiol 1973;232:331–356.
11 Diamond DM, Weinberger NM: Classical conditioning rapidly induces specific changes in frequency receptive fields of single neurons in secondary and ventral ectosylvian auditory cortical fields. Brain Res 1986;372:357–360.

12 Weinberger NM, Diamond DM: Physiological plasticity in auditory cortex: rapid induction by learning. Prog Neurobiol 1987;29:1–55.

13 Robertson D, Irvine DRF: Plasticity of frequency organization in auditory cortex of guinea pigs with partial unilateral deafness. J Comp Neurol 1989;282:456–471.

14 Snyder RL, Sinex DG, McGee JD, Walsh EW: Acute spiral ganglion lesions change the tuning and tonotopic organization of cat inferior colliculus neurons. Hear Res 2000;147:200–220.

15 Snyder RL, Sinex DG: Immediate changes in tuning of inferior colliculus neurons following acute lesions of cat spiral ganglion. J Neurophysiol 2002;87:434–452.

16 Recanzone GH, Schreiner CE, Merzenich MM: Plasticity in the frequency representation of primary auditory cortex following discrimination training in adult owl monkeys. J Neurosci 1993;13:87–103.

17 Harrison RV, Stanton SG, Mount RJ: Effects of chronic cochlear damage on threshold and frequency tuning of neurons in AI auditory cortex. Acta Otolaryngol Suppl 1995;519:30–35.

18 Stanton SG, Harrison RV: Abnormal cochleotopic organization in the auditory cortex of cats reared in a frequency augmented environment. Auditory Neurosci 1996;2:97–107.

19 Kilgard MP, Pandya PK, Vazquez J, Gehi A, Schreiner CE, Merzenich MM: Sensory input directs spatial and temporal plasticity in primary auditory cortex. J Neurophysiol 2001;86:326–338.

20 Bakin JS, Lepan B, Weinberger NM: Sensitization induced receptive field plasticity in the auditory cortex is independent of CS-modality. Brain Res 1992;577:226–235.

21 Edeline JM, Pham P, Weinberger NM: Rapid development of learning-induced receptive field plasticity in the auditory cortex. Behav Neurosci 1993;107:539–551.

22 Edeline JM, Weinberger NM: Receptive field plasticity in the auditory cortex during frequency discrimination training: selective retuning independent of task difficulty. Behav Neurosci 1993;107:82–103.

23 Weinberger NM: Tuning the brain by leaning and by stimulation of the nucleus basalis. Trends Cogn Sci 1998;2:271–273.

24 Pandya PK, Moucha R, Engineer ND, Rathbun DL, Vazquez J, Kilgard MP: Asynchronous inputs alter excitability, spike timing, and topography in primary auditory cortex. Hear Res 2005;203:10–20.

25 Kilgard MP, Merzenich MM: Plasticity of temporal information processing in the primary auditory cortex. Nat Neurosci 1998;1:727–731.

26 Suga N, Ma XF: Multiparametric corticofugal modulation and plasticity in the auditory system. Nat Rev Neurosci 2003;4:783–794.

27 Juliano SL: Mapping the sensory mosaic. Science 1998;279:1653–1654.

28 Kamke MR, Brown M, Irvine DR: Basal forebrain cholinergic input is not essential for lesion-induced plasticity in mature auditory cortex. Neuron 2005;48:675–686.

29 Kilgard MP: Cortical Map Reorganization without Cholinergic Modulation. Neuron 2005;48:529–530.

30 Diamond DM, Weinberger NM: Physiological plasticity of single neurons in auditory cortex of the cat during acquisition of the pupillary conditioned response: II. Secondary field AII. Behav Neurosci 1984;98:189–210.

31 Ferrer I, Soriano E, Del Rio JA, Alcantara S, Auladell C: Cell death and removal in the cerebral cortex during development. Prog Neurobiol 1992;39:1–43.

32 Oppenheim RW: Cell death during development of the nervous system. Annu Rev Neurosci 1991;14:453–501.

33 Conel JL: The Postnatal Development of Human Cerebral Cortex. Vol. I–VIII. Cambridge MA: Harvard University Press, 1939–1967.

34 Cragg BG: The development of synapses in kitten visual cortex during visual deprivation. Exp Neurol 1975;46:445–451.

35 Winfield DA: The postnatal development of synapses in the different laminae of the visual cortex in the normal kitten and in kittens with eyelid suture. Brain Res 1983;285:155–169.

36 O'Kusky JR: Synapse elimination in the developing visual cortex: a morphometric analysis in normal and dark-reared cats. Brain Res 1985;354:81–91.

37 Huttenlocher PR, Dabholkar AS: Regional differences in synaptogenesis in human cerebral cortex. J Comp Neurol 1997;387:167–178.

38   Payne BR: Development of the auditory cortex; in Romand R (ed): Development of Auditory and Vestibular Systems 2. Amsterdam, Elsevier Science Publishers B.V., 1992, pp 357–390.

39   Harrison RV, Nagasawa A, Smith DW, Stanton S, Mount RJ: Reorganization of auditory cortex after neonatal high frequency cochlear hearing loss. Hear Res 1991;54:11–19.

40   Ramus F, Hauser MD, Miller C, Morris D, Mehler J: Language discrimination by human newborns and by cotton-top tamarin monkeys. Science 2000;288:349–351.

41   Locke JL: A theory of neurolinguistic development. Brain Lang 1997;58:265–326.

42   Dehaene-Lambertz G, Dehaene S, Hertz-Pannier L: Functional neuroimaging of speech perception in infants. Science 2002;298:2013–2015.

43   Pena M, Maki A, Kovacic D, DehaeneLambertz G, Koizumi H, Bouquet F, et al: Sounds and silence: an optical topography study of language recognition at birth. Proc Natl Acad Sci USA 2003;100:11702–11705.

44   Winkler I, Kushnerenko E, Horvath J, Ceponiene R, Fellman V, Huotilainen M, et al: Newborn infants can organize the auditory world. Proc Natl Acad Sci USA 2003;100:11812–11815.

45   Werker JF, Tees RC: Developmental changes across childhood in the perception of non-native speech sounds. Can J Psychol 1983;37:278–286.

46   Werker JF, Tees RC: Cross-language speech perception: evidence for perceptual reorganization during the first year of life. Infant Behav Dev 1984;7:49–63.

47   Kuhl PK: Early language acquisition: cracking the speech code. Nat Rev Neurosci 2004;5: 831–843.

48   Ruben RJ: A time frame of critical/sensitive periods of language development. Acta Otolaryngol 1997;117:202–205.

49   Kral A, Tillein J, Heid S, Hartmann R, Klinke R: Postnatal cortical development in congenital auditory deprivation. Cereb Cortex 2005;15:552–562.

50   Kral A, Hartmann R, Tillein J, Heid S, Klinke R: Delayed maturation and sensitive periods in the auditory cortex. Audiol Neurootol 2001;6:346–362.

51   Syka J: Plastic changes in the central auditory system after hearing loss, restoration of function, and during learning. Physiol Rev 2002;82:601–636.

52   Calford MB: Dynamic representational plasticity in sensory cortex. Neuroscience 2002;111: 709–738.

53   Pascual-Leone A, Amedi A, Fregni F, Merabet LB: The plastic human brain cortex. Annu Rev Neurosci 2005;28:377–401.

54   Pascalis O, Scott LS, Kelly DJ, Shannon RW, Nicholson E, Coleman M, et al: Plasticity of face processing in infancy. Proc Natl Acad Sci USA 2005;102:5297–5300.

55   Moller AR: Neural plasticity and disorders of the nervous system. Cambridge, Cambridge University Press, 2006.

56   Hartmann R, Kral A: Central responses to electrical stimulation; in Zeng FG, Popper AN, Fay RR (eds): Cochlear Implants: Auditory Prostheses and Electric Hearing. New York, Springer, 2004, pp 213–285.

57   Kitzes LM, Kageyama GH, Semple MN, Kil J: Development of ectopic projections from the ventral cochlear nucleus to the superior olivary complex induced by neonatal ablation of the contralateral cochlea. J Comp Neurol 1995;353:341–363.

58   Russell FA, Moore DR: Effects of unilateral cochlear removal on dendrites in the gerbil medial superior olivary nucleus. Eur J Neurosci 1999;11:1379–1390.

59   Leake-Jones PA, Vivion MC, O'Reilly BF, Merzenich MM: Deaf animal models for studies of a multichannel cochlear prosthesis. Hear Res 1982;8:225–246.

60   Xu S-A, Shepherd RK, Chen Y, Clark GM: Profound hearing loss in the cat following the single co-administration of kanamycin and ethacrynic acid. Hear Res 1993;70:205–215.

61   Niparko JK, Finger PA: Cochlear nucleus cell size changes in the dalmatian: model of congenital deafness. Otolaryngol Head Neck Surg 1997;117:229–235.

62   Larsen SA, Kirchhoff TM: Anatomical evidence of synaptic plasticity in the cochlear nuclei of white-deaf cats. Exp Neurol 1992;115:151–157.

63   Heid S, Hartmann R, Klinke R: A model for prelingual deafness, the congenitally deaf white cat – population statistics and degenerative changes. Hear Res 1998;115:101–112.

64   Mair IWS: Hereditary deafness in the white cat. Acta Otolaryngol Stockh 1973;314(suppl):1–53.

65   Tierney TS, Moore DR: Naturally occurring neuron death during postnatal development of the gerbil ventral cochlear nucleus begins at the onset of hearing. J Comp Neurol 1997;387: 421–429.

66   Mostafapour SP, Del Puerto NM, Rubel EW: bcl-2 Overexpression eliminates deprivation-induced cell death of brainstem auditory neurons. J Neurosci 2002;22:4670–4674.

67   Pasic TR, Rubel EW: Rapid changes in cochlear nucleus cell size following blockade of auditory nerve electrical activity in gerbils. J Comp Neurol 1989;283:474–480.

68   Morest DK, Bohne BA: Noise-induced degeneration in the brain and representation of inner and outer hair cells. Hear Res 1983;9:145–152.

69   Nordeen KW, Killackey HP, Kitzes LM: Ascending projections to the inferior colliculus following unilateral cochlear ablation in the neonatal gerbil, Meriones unguiculatus. J Comp Neurol 1983; 214:144–153.

70   Heid S: Morphologische Befunde am peripheren und zentralen auditorischen System der kongenital gehörlosen weißen Katze. Frankfurt am Main, J.W. Goethe University, 1998.

71   Hardie NA, Martsi-McClintock A, Aitkin LM, Shepherd RK: Neonatal sensorineural hearing loss affects synaptic density in the auditory midbrain. Neuroreport 1998;9:2019–2022.

72   Hardie NA, Shepherd RK: Sensorineural hearing loss during development: morphological and physiological response of the cochlea and auditory brainstem. Hear Res 1999;128:147–165.

73   Ryugo DK, Rosenbaum BT, Kim PJ, Niparko JK, Saada AA: Single unit recordings in the auditory nerve of congenitally deaf white cats: morphological correlates in the cochlea and cochlear nucleus. J Comp Neurol 1998;397:532–548.

74   Moore JK, Niparko JK, Perazzo LM, Miller MR, Linthicum FH: Effect of adult-onset deafness on the human central auditory system. Ann Otol Rhinol Laryngol 1997;106:385–390.

75   Ryugo DK, Kretzmer EA, Niparko JK: Restoration of auditory nerve synapses in cats by cochlear implants. Science 2005;310:1490–1492.

76   Snyder RL, Rebscher SJ, Leake PA, Kelly K, Cao K: Chronic intracochlear electrical stimulation in the neonatally deafened cat. 2. Temporal properties of neurons in the inferior colliculus. Hear Res 1991;56:246–264.

77   Klinke R, Kral A, Heid S, Tillein J, Hartmann R: Recruitment of the auditory cortex in congenitally deaf cats by long-term cochlear electrostimulation. Science 1999;285:1729–1733.

78   Kral A, Hartmann R, Tillein J, Heid S, Klinke R: Hearing after congenital deafness: central auditory plasticity and sensory deprivation. Cereb Cortex 2002;12:797–807.

79   Snyder RL, Rebscher SJ, Cao K, Leake PA, Kelly K: Chronic intracochlear electrical stimulation in the neonatally deafened cat. 1. Expansion of central representation. Hear Res 1990;50:7–34.

80   Shepherd RK, Baxi JH, Hardie NA: Response of inferior colliculus neurons to electrical stimulation of the auditory nerve in neonatally deafened cats. J Neurophysiol 1999;82:1363–1380.

81   Heid S, Jahnsiebert TK, Klinke R, Hartmann R, Langner G: Afferent projection patterns in the auditory brainstem in normal and congenitally deaf white cats. Hear Res 1997;110:191–199.

82   Bledsoe SC, Nagase S, Miller JM, Altschuler RA: Deafness-induced plasticity in the mature central auditory system. Neuroreport 1995;7:225–229.

83   Vale C, Sanes DH: Afferent regulation of inhibitory synaptic transmission in the developing auditory midbrain. J Neurosci 2000;20:1912–1921.

84   Gordon KA, Papsin BC, Harrison RV: Auditory brain stem and midbrain development after cochlear implantation in children. Ann Otol Rhinol Laryngol Suppl 2002;189:32–37.

85   Snyder R, Leake P, Rebscher S, Beitel R: Temporal resolution of neurons in cat inferior colliculus to intracochlear electrical stimulation: effects of neonatal deafening and chronic stimulation. J Neurophysiol 1995;73:449–467.

86   Vollmer M, Snyder RL, Leake PA, Beitel RE, Moore CM, Rebscher SJ: Temporal properties of chronic cochlear electrical stimulation determine temporal resolution of neurons in cat inferior colliculus. J Neurophysiol 1999;82:2883–2902.

87   Moore CM, Vollmer M, Leake PA, Snyder RL, Rebscher SJ: The effects of chronic intracochlear electrical stimulation on inferior colliculus spatial representation in adult deafened cats. Hear Res 2002;164:82–96.

88   Kral A, Schroder JH, Klinke R, Engel AK: Absence of cross-modal reorganization in the primary auditory cortex of congenitally deaf cats. Exp Brain Res 2003;153:605–613.

89 Raggio MW, Schreiner CE: Neuronal responses in cat primary auditory cortex to electrical cochlear stimulation. 1. Intensity dependence of firing rate and response latency. J Neurophysiol 1994;72:2334–2359.

90 Hartmann R, Shepherd RK, Heid S, Klinke R: Response of the primary auditory cortex to electrical stimulation of the auditory nerve in the congenitally deaf white cat. Hear Res 1997;112:115–133.

91 Bavelier D, Neville HJ: Cross-modal plasticity: where and how? Nat Rev Neurosci 2002;3:443–452.

92 Stanton SG, Harrison RV: Projections from the medial geniculate body to primary auditory cortex in neonatally deafened cats. J Comp Neurol 2000;426:117–129.

93 Raggio MW, Schreiner CE: Neuronal responses in cat primary auditory cortex to electrical cochlear stimulation. III. Activation patterns in short- and long-term deafness. J Neurophysiol 1999;82:3506–3526.

94 Kral A, Hartmann R, Tillein J, Heid S, Klinke R: Congenital auditory deprivation reduces synaptic activity within the auditory cortex in a layer-specific manner. Cereb Cortex 2000;10:714–726.

95 Larkum ME, Zhu JJ, Sakmann B: A new cellular mechanism for coupling inputs arriving at different cortical layers. Nature 1999;398:338–341.

96 Feldmeyer D, Sakmann B: Synaptic efficacy and reliability of excitatory connections between the principal neurones of the input layer 4 and output layer 5 of the neocortex. J Physiol 2000;525:31–39.

97 de Ribaupierre F: Acoustic information processing in the auditory thalamus and cerebral cortex; in Ehret G, Romand R (eds): The Central Auditory System. New York, Oxford, Oxford University Press, 1997, pp 317–397.

98 Raizada RDS, Grossberg S: Towards a theory of the laminar architecture of cerebral cortex: computational clues from the visual system. Cereb Cortex 2003;13:100–113.

99 Kaczmarek L, Kossut M, Skangiel-Kramska J: Glutamate receptors in cortical plasticity: molecular and cellular biology. Physiol Rev 1997;77:217–255.

100 Fryauf-Bertschy H, Tyler RS, Kelsay DM, Gantz BJ, Woodworth GG: Cochlear implant use by prelingually deafened children: the influences of age at implant and length of device use. J Speech Lang Hear Res 1997;40:183–199.

101 Moore CM, Vollmer M, Leake PA, Snyder RL, Rebscher SJ: The effects of chronic intracochlear electrical stimulation on inferior colliculus spatial representation in adult deafened cats. Hear Res 2002;164:82–96.

102 Gordon KA, Papsin BC, Harrison RV: An evoked potential study of the developmental time course of the auditory nerve and brainstem in children using cochlear implants. Audiol Neurootol 2006;11:7–23.

103 Winfield DA: The postnatal development of synapses in the visual cortex of the cat and the effects of eyelid closure. Brain Res 1981;206:166–171.

104 Sharma A, Dorman And MF, Spahr AJ: A sensitive period for the development of the central auditory system in children with cochlear implants: implications for age of implantation. Ear Hear 2002;23:532–539.

105 Sharma A, Dorman MF, Spahr AJ: Rapid development of cortical auditory evoked potentials after early cochlear implantation. Neuroreport 2002;13:1365–1368.

106 Sharma A, Dorman MF, Kral A: The influence of a sensitive period on central auditory development in children with unilateral and bilateral cochlear implants. Hear Res 2005;203:134–143.

107 Gordon KA, Papsin BC, Harrison RV: Effects of cochlear implant use on the electrically evoked middle latency response in children. Hear Res 2005;204:78–89.

108 Pallas SL, Littman T, Moore DR: Cross-modal reorganization of callosal connectivity without altering thalamocortical projections. Proc Natl Acad Sci USA 1999;96:8751–8756.

109 Pallas SL, Sur M: Visual projections induced into the auditory pathway of ferrets. II. Corticocortical connections of primary auditory cortex. J Comp Neurol 1993;337:317–333.

110 Pallas SL, Roe AW, Sur M: Visual projections induced into the auditory pathway of ferrets. I. Novel inputs to primary auditory cortex AI from the LP/pulvinar complex and the topography of the MGN-AI projection. J Comp Neurol 1990;298:50–68.

111 von Melchner L, Pallas SL, Sur M: Visual behaviour mediated by retinal projections directed to the auditory pathway. Nature 2000;404:871–876.

112 Wakita M, Watanabe S: Compensatory plasticity following neonatal lesion of the auditory cortex. Biomed Res 1997;18:79–89.

113 Møller AR: Hearing: Its Physiology and Pathophysiology. Amsterdam, Elsevier Science, 2006.

114 Møller AR, Rollins PR: The non-classical auditory pathways are involved in hearing in children but not in adults. Neurosci Lett 2002;319:41–44.

115 Møller AR, Møller MB, Yokota M: Some forms of tinnitus may involve the extralemniscal auditory pathway. Laryngoscope 1992;102:1165–1171.

116 Nishimura H, Hashikawa K, Doi K, Iwaki T, Watanabe Y, Kusuoka H, et al: Sign language 'heard' in the auditory cortex. Nature 1999;397:116.

117 Petitto LA, Zatorre RJ, Gauna K, Nikelski EJ, Dostie D, Evans AC: Speech-like cerebral activity in profoundly deaf people processing signed languages: implications for the neural basis of human language. Proc Natl Acad Sci USA 2000;97:13961–13966.

118 Finney EM, Fine I, Dobkins KR: Visual stimuli activate auditory cortex in the deaf. Nat Neurosci 2001;4:1171–1173.

119 Lee DS, Lee JS, Oh SH, Kim SK, Kim JW, Chung JK, et al: Cross-modal plasticity and cochlear implants. Nature 2001;409:149–150.

120 Bernstein LE, Auer ET, Moore JK, Ponton CW, Don M, Singh M: Visual speech perception without primary auditory cortex activation. Neuroreport 2002;13:311–315.

121 Stewart DL, Starr A: Absence of visually influenced cells in auditory cortex of normal and congenitally deaf cats. Exp Neurol 1970;28:525–528.

122 Naito Y, Okazawa H, Honjo I, Hirano S, Takahashi H, Shiomi Y, et al: Cortical activation with sound stimulation in cochlear implant users demonstrated by positron emission tomography. Brain Res Cogn Brain Res 1995;2:207–214.

123 Naito Y, Hirano S, Honjo I, Okazawa H, Ishizu K, Takahashi H, et al: Sound-induced activation of auditory cortices in cochlear implant users with post- and prelingual deafness demonstrated by positron emission tomography. Acta Otolaryngol 1997;117:490–496.

Professor A. Kral, MD, PhD
Institute of Neurophysiology and Pathophysiology
Martinistrasse 52
DE–20246 Hamburg (Germany)
Tel. +49 40 42803 7046, Fax +49 40 42803 7752, E-Mail a.kral@uke.uni-hamburg.de

Møller AR (ed): Cochlear and Brainstem Implants.
Adv Otorhinolaryngol. Basel, Karger, 2006, vol 64, pp 109–143

Speech Processing in Vocoder-Centric Cochlear Implants

Philipos C. Loizou

Department of Electrical Engineering, Jonsson School of Engineering and Computer
Science, University of Texas at Dallas, Richardson, Tex., USA

Abstract

The principles of the most recent cochlear implant processors are similar to that of the
channel vocoder, originally used for transmitting speech over telephone lines with much less
bandwidth than that required for transmitting the unprocessed speech signal. An overview of
the various vocoder-centric processing strategies proposed for cochlear implants since the late
1990s is provided including the strategies used in different commercially available implant
processors. Special emphasis is placed on reviewing the strategies designed to enhance pitch
information for potentially better music perception. The various noise suppression strategies
proposed over the years based on multi-microphone and single-microphone inputs are also
described.

This paper presents an overview of the various vocoder-centric processing strategies proposed for cochlear implants (CIs) since the late 1990s [for a review of earlier strategies, see 1]. This paper also offers a review of the strategies used in different commercially available implant processors.

Historical Background

In 1939, at the World's Fair in New York City, people watched with intense curiosity the first talking machine. The machine spoke with the help of a human operator seating in front of a console, similar to a piano keyboard, consisting of 10 keys, a pedal and a wrist bar. Inside the machine were analog circuits of band-pass filters, switches and amplifiers connected to a loudspeaker. The talking machine contained the first artificial speech-synthesis system implemented

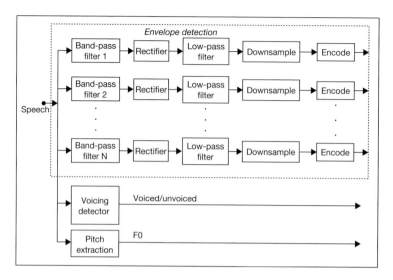

Fig. 1. The channel vocoder analyzer. The signal processing blocks enclosed in the dashed rectangle are used in most cochlear implant devices.

in hardware. This speech synthesis system, pioneered by Homer Dudley from Bell Laboratories, came to be known as the channel vocoder (voice coder) [2]. Dudley's vocoder idea had a profound impact not only on telephony and speech transmission applications [3, 4], but also much later in the development of CI processors. The latest and most successful signal-processing strategies used in CIs are based on vocoding analysis principles. All CI devices today are programmed (now digitally) with a modified version of the vocoder analysis algorithm.

The Channel Vocoder

The channel vocoder [2, 4] consists of a speech analyzer and a speech synthesizer (figs. 1 and 2). In speech transmission applications, the analyzer would be utilized at the transmitter and the synthesizer at the receiver end. The incoming signal is first filtered into a number of contiguous frequency channels using a bank of band-pass filters (10 filters were used in Dudley's 1939 demonstration). The envelope of the signal in each channel is estimated by full-wave rectification and low-pass filtering and is then downsampled and quantized for transmission. In addition to envelope estimation, the vocoder analyzer makes a voiced/unvoiced decision and estimates the vocal pitch (F0) of the signal. These

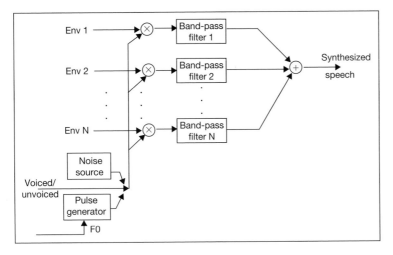

Fig. 2. The channel vocoder synthesizer.

two pieces of information are transmitted alongside the envelope information. The synthesizer modulates the received envelopes by the appropriate excitation as determined by the voiced/unvoiced (binary) signal. The excitation signal consists of random noise for unvoiced speech segments and a periodic pulse generator for voiced speech, with the period of the pulse generator being controlled by F0. The modulated signals are subsequently band-pass-filtered by the same filters and then added together to produce the synthesized speech waveform.

Current CI processors (60 years later) utilize the same blocks of the channel vocoder analyzer shown in figure 1. At present, only the vocoder analyzer is used for transmitting envelope information to the individual electrodes, but recently there has been a shift in research focus toward implementing blocks of the synthesizer as well [5, 6]. Interestingly, early devices based on feature extraction strategies modulated the estimated formant amplitudes by F0 [1]. These strategies, however, were abandoned due to the inherent difficulties associated with F0 extraction in noisy environments. It is also interesting to note that the acoustic CI simulations often used to study performance of CI patients in the absence of confounding factors (e.g. duration of deafness, insertion depth) utilize the synthesizer (fig. 2). By choosing random noise as the excitation signals for all segments of speech, we get the noise-band CI simulations [7]. Similarly, by choosing sine waves with frequencies set to the center frequencies of the band-pass filters as the excitation signals, we get the sine wave simulations [8].

Vocoder-Centric Strategies for Cochlear Implants

There are currently two variations of the channel vocoder (fig. 1) that are used in all implant processors. The first implementation uses the analyzer of the channel vocoder in its original form (fig. 1). The second implementation also uses the analyzer of the channel vocoder, but selects only a subset of the envelope outputs for stimulation. This section describes in detail these two variations.

Continuous Interleaved Sampling Strategy

The first device to adopt a channel-vocoder strategy was the Ineraid device manufactured by Symbion, Inc., Utah. The signal was first compressed using an automatic gain control, and then filtered into four contiguous frequency bands, with center frequencies at 0.5, 1, 2, and 3.4 kHz [9]. The filtered waveforms went through adjustable gain controls and were then sent directly through a percutaneous connection to four intracochlear electrodes. The filtered waveforms were delivered simultaneously to four electrodes in analog form. A major concern associated with simultaneous stimulation is the interaction between channels caused by the summation of electrical fields from individual electrodes. Neural responses to stimuli from one electrode may be significantly distorted by stimuli from other electrodes. These interactions may distort speech spectral information and therefore degrade speech understanding.

A simple solution to the channel interaction problem was proposed by researchers at the Research Triangle Institute via the use of nonsimultaneous, interleaved pulses [10]. They proposed modulating the filtered waveforms by trains of biphasic pulses that were delivered to the electrodes in a nonoverlapping (nonsimultaneous) fashion, that is, in a way such that only one electrode was stimulated at a time (fig. 3). The amplitudes of the pulses were derived by extracting the envelopes of the band-passed waveforms. The resulting strategy was called the continuous interleaved sampling (CIS) strategy.

The block diagram of the CIS strategy is shown in figure 3. The signal is first pre-emphasized and then applied to a bank of band-pass filters. The envelopes of the outputs of these band-pass filters are then full-wave rectified and low-pass filtered (typically with 200- or 400-Hz cutoff frequency). The envelopes of the outputs of the band-pass filters are finally compressed and used to modulate biphasic pulses. A nonlinear compression function (e.g. logarithmic) is used to ensure that the envelope outputs fit the patient's dynamic range of electrically evoked hearing. Trains of balanced biphasic pulses, with amplitudes proportional to the envelopes, are delivered to the electrodes at a constant rate in a nonoverlapping fashion.

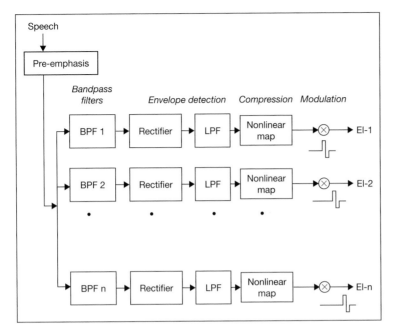

Fig. 3. Block diagram of the signal processing involved in the CIS strategy. BPF = Band-pass filter; LPF = low-pass filter.

Figure 3 shows the basic configuration for the CIS strategy. Many variations of the CIS strategy have emerged and are currently used by the three implant manufacturers. Some devices, for instance, use the fast Fourier transform (FFT) for spectral analysis, and some use the Hilbert transform to extract the envelope instead of full-wave rectification and low-pass filtering. Although the CIS strategy is employed by all three manufacturers, it is based on different implementations.

CIS Design Parameters

The CIS strategy can be configured in a number of ways by varying design parameters (e.g. filter spacing, envelope cut-off frequencies, etc.) of the vocoder. These parameters include, among other things, the envelope detection method, stimulation rate (i.e. the number of pulses delivered to the electrodes per second), shape of compression function and filter spacing. A subset of these parameters may be varied to optimize speech recognition performance for each patient.

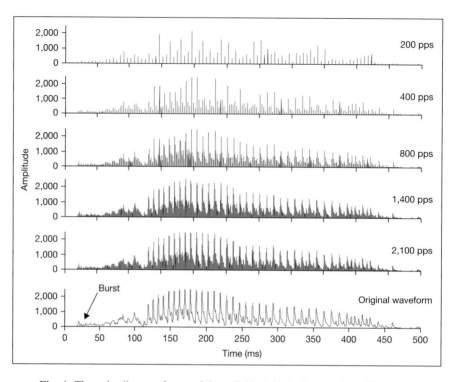

Fig. 4. The pulsatile waveforms of the syllable /t i/ obtained at five different stimulation rates [12]. These waveforms were obtained by band-pass filtering the syllable /t i/ into 6 channels, performing envelope detection, and sampling the rectified envelopes at the rates indicated. Only the waveforms for channel 5 (with a center frequency of 3,316 Hz) are shown. The bottom panel shows the original speech envelopes of channel 5. This figure shows the effect of stimulation rate in detecting short-duration segments (e.g. burst) of speech. As the pulse rate increases, the burst becomes more distinctive, and perhaps more salient perceptually. Reprinted with permission from Loizou et al. [12].

Stimulation Rate

The pulse rate – the number of pulses per second (pps) delivered to each electrode – may be as low as 250 pps or as high as 5,000 pps in some devices. It is reasonable to expect that better recognition performance should be obtained with high pulse rates, since high pulse rate stimulation can better represent fine temporal modulations. This is illustrated in figure 4, which shows the pulsatile waveforms of the syllable /t i/ obtained at different rates. As shown in figure 4, the unvoiced stop consonant /t/ is marked by a period of silence (closure) followed by a burst and aspiration. As the pulse rate increases, the burst becomes more distinctive, and perhaps more salient perceptually. There seems to be no evidence of the burst at low rates, 200 or 400 pps. This example clearly demonstrates that lower rates do not provide a good, if any at all, temporal representation of the burst in stop consonants.

Despite the theoretical advantages of higher stimulation rates, the outcomes from several studies have not been consistent. While the majority of those studies [11–15] found a positive effect of high stimulation rates, a few studies [16, 17] found no significant effect. It is, however, consistent across these studies that some patients received large benefits with high stimulation rates while other patients received, little, or no benefit. Possible reasons for the discrepancies in the outcomes between the various studies include: (a) differences in implementation of the CIS strategy, (b) differences in speech materials used, and (c) differences in electrode design between devices. Each manufacturer has its own implementation of the CIS strategy. In the Nucleus device, for instance, the FFT is used for spectral analysis in lieu of the bank of band-pass filters. Limited by the FFT analysis frame rate, extremely high stimulation rates can be obtained by repeating stimulus frames. Therefore, higher stimulation rates might not necessarily introduce new information, which explains the lack of improvement with high stimulation rates [16].

The influence of speech materials when examining the effect of parametric variations of the CIS strategy was demonstrated in the study by Loizou et al. [12], which assessed speech recognition as a function of stimulation rate in six Med-El/CIS-Link CI listeners. Results showed that higher stimulation rates >2,100 pps produced a significantly higher performance on word and consonant recognition than lower stimulation rates (800 pps). The effect of stimulation rate on consonant recognition was highly dependent on the vowel context. The largest benefit was noted for consonants in the /iCi/ and /uCu/ contexts, while the smallest benefit was noted for consonants in the /aCa/ context. This finding suggests that the /aCa/ consonant test, which is widely used, is not sensitive enough to parametric variations of implant processors.

The advantages of high stimulation rates are unfortunately offset by the increased channel interaction concomitant with extremely high stimulation rates. Each manufacturer uses a different number of electrode contacts with different electrode spacing (table 1). It is reasonable to assume that a wider spacing between electrodes will yield smaller amounts of channel interaction. Consequently, the electrode spacing confounds the effect of high stimulation rates on speech recognition when comparing different devices. The Nucleus device has the smallest electrode spacing (0.7 mm), while the Med-El device has the widest electrode spacing (2.4 mm). The Ineraid device has in fact the widest spacing (4 mm), but is not commercially available. It is therefore not surprising that most of the benefits reported with high stimulation rates were with Med-El users and not with Nucleus users. Significant benefits were reported in studies by Skinner

Table 1. Characteristics of commercially available cochlear implant devices

Device	Processor name	Electrodes		Stimulation
		number	spacing, mm	
Nucleus	ESPrit/Freedom	22	0.7	sequential
Clarion II	Auria	16	1.1	sequential/simultaneous
Med-El	COMBI40+/ Tempo+/ PULSARci[100]	12	2.4	sequential/simultaneous[1]

[1]Supported only in the PULSARci[100] processor.

et al. [15] and Kim et al. [18] with Nucleus users, but with those users fitted with a spectral-maxima strategy running at high stimulation rates.

As mentioned above, some patients do receive significant benefit with the use of high stimulation rates. The 'optimal' pulse rate, however, as far as speech recognition performance is concerned, varies from patient to patient. Wilson et al. [11], for instance, reported that some patients obtain a maximum performance on the 16-consonant recognition task with a pulse rate of 833 pps and pulse duration of 33 μs/phase. Other patients obtain small but significant increases in performance as the pulse rate is increased from 833 to 1,365 pps, and from 1,365 to 2,525 pps, using 33 μs/phase pulses. Unfortunately, there are no known methods for identifying the 'optimal' pulse rate for each patient, other than trying out different values and examining their performance.

Current commercial implant processors are operating at stimulation rates ranging from 800 pps/channel to 2,500 pps/channel, depending on the device. Use of very high rates (>5,000 pps) is being investigated by some as a means of restoring the stochastic independence of neural responses, which is lost with the overly synchronized electrical stimulation. In acoustic hearing, it is known that the nature of the neuron responses is stochastic in that the firing of a particular auditory nerve fiber has no effect on the probability of a neighboring fiber firing. In electric stimulation, however, the response of single neurons is highly synchronized and also entrained with the stimulus, in that neurons fire on every stimulation cycle, up to the rates of 800 Hz [19, 20]. The stochastic nature (i.e. the independence) of the neural responses is lost with electrical stimulation since all the neurons in a local region fire at the same time (i.e., in synchrony). To restore the stochastic independence of neuron responses, Rubinstein et al. [21] proposed the use of high-frequency (5,000 pps) desynchronizing pulse trains over the stimulus delivered by the processor. Litvak et al. [22] demonstrated that the use of desynchronizing pulse trains can improve the representation of both sinusoidal and complex stimuli (synthetic vowels) in the temporal discharge patterns of auditory nerve fibers for frequencies up to 1,000 Hz. The addition of unmodulated high-rate pulse trains over the electrical stimulus can also result in significant increases in psychophysical dynamic range [23]. Another method proposed for restoring the stochastic independence of neural responses is the addition of appropriate amount of noise to the acoustic stimuli [24, 25].

Compression Function

The compression of envelope amplitudes is an essential component of the CIS processor because it transforms acoustical amplitudes into electrical amplitudes. This transformation is necessary because the range in acoustic amplitudes in conversational speech is considerably larger than the implant patient's dynamic range. Dynamic range is defined here as the range in electrical amplitudes between threshold (barely audible level) and uncomfortable loudness level (extremely loud). In conversational speech, the acoustic amplitudes may vary within a range of 30–50 dB [26, 27]. Implant listeners, however, may have a dynamic range as small as 5 dB. For that reason, the CIS processor compresses, using a nonlinear compression function, the acoustic amplitudes to fit the patient's electrical dynamic range. The logarithmic function is commonly used for compression because it matches the loudness between acoustic and electrical amplitudes [28, 29]. It has been shown that the loudness of an electrical stimulus in microamps is analogous to the loudness of an acoustic stimulus in dB.

Logarithmic compression functions of the form $Y = A \log(1+CX) + B$ are typically used, where X is the acoustic amplitude (output of envelope detector), A, B and C are constants, and Y is the (compressed) electrical amplitude. Other types of compression functions used are the power-law functions of the form:

$$y = Ax^p + B \tag{1}$$

where $p < 1$. The advantage of using power-law functions is that the shape, and particularly the steepness of the compression function, can be easily controlled by simply varying the value of the exponent p. The constants A and B are chosen such that the input acoustic range is mapped to the electrical dynamic range (THR, MCL), where THR is the threshold level and MCL is the most comfortable level measured in μA [1]. The input acoustic range, also known as input dynamic range, is adjustable in some devices and can range from 30 to 70 dB. The effect of input dynamic range on speech recognition was examined in several studies [e.g. 27, 30].

The effect of the shape of the compression function on speech recognition has been investigated in a number of studies [12, 31–34]. Loizou et al. [12]

modified the shape of the amplitude mapping functions ranging from strongly compressive to weakly compressive by varying the power exponent in equation (1) from p = −0.1 (too compressive) to p = 0.5 (nearly linear). Results indicated that the shape of the compression function had only a minor effect on performance, with the lowest performance obtained for nearly linear mapping functions.

Envelope Detection

Two different methods can be used to extract the envelopes of filtered waveforms. The first method includes rectification (full-wave or half-wave) followed by low-pass filtering at 200–400 Hz. The second method, currently used by the Med-El device, uses the Hilbert transform. No clear advantage has been demonstrated for the use of one method over the other for envelope extraction.

The first method is simple to implement as it involves full-wave or half-wave rectification and low-pass filtering. The low-pass filter is a smoothing filter and also serves as an antialiasing filter, which is required prior to downsampling (fig. 1) the filtered waveforms. The stimulation rate needs to be at least two times higher (Nyquist rate) than the cutoff-frequency of the low-pass filter. Psychophysics studies [35] suggest that it should be at least four times the envelope cutoff frequency. Pitch increased with sinusoidally amplitude-modulated pulse trains up to a modulation frequency of about 200–300 Hz, provided the carrier rate (stimulation rate) was at least four times the modulation frequency [35]. Similar findings were also reported in intracochlear evoked potential studies [36].

The cut-off frequency of the low-pass filter controls the modulation depth of the envelopes. The lower the cutoff frequency is, the smaller the modulation depth of the filtered waveform (see fig. 7), i.e. the flatter the envelopes are. Simulation studies [7, 37] demonstrated no significant effect of the envelope cutoff frequency on speech recognition by normal-hearing listeners. This was also confirmed with studies from our lab with CI patients (fig. 5) tested on consonant and melody recognition tasks [38]. No significant effect of envelope cutoff frequency on consonant and melody recognition was found.

The second envelope detection method is based on the Hilbert transform [39], a mathematical tool which can represent a time waveform as a product of slowly-varying envelope and a 'carrier' signal, containing fine structure information (fig. 6). More specifically, the filtered waveform, $x_i(t)$, in the ith band (channel) can be represented as

$$x_i(t) = a_i(t) \cos f_i(t) \tag{2}$$

where $a_i(t)$ represents the envelope of the ith band at time t, and $\cos[f_i(t)]$ represents the fine-structure waveform of the ith band. Note that $f_i(t)$ is called the instantaneous phase of the signal, and the derivative of $f_i(t)$ produces the instantaneous frequency (carrier frequency) of the signal, which varies over time. The

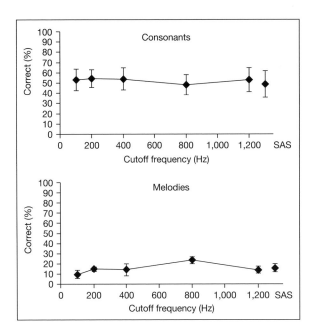

Fig. 5. Consonant and familiar melody identification as a function of envelope cutoff frequency (Hz). Plots show mean identification scores (% correct) for 5 Clarion-S users fitted with the SAS strategy. Error bars indicate standard errors of the mean. The melodies were taken from a set of 34 simple melodies with all rhythmic information removed [116] and consisted of 16 equal-duration notes synthesized using samples of a grand piano. Prior to the melody recognition test, the subjects selected ten melodies (e.g. 'Twinkle Twinkle', 'Old McDonald') that they were familiar with. The consonant test included 16 consonants in /aCa/ format produced by a male speaker.

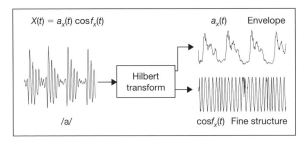

Fig. 6. Decomposition of a signal (taken from the vowel /a/) into its envelope and fine structure using the Hilbert transform.

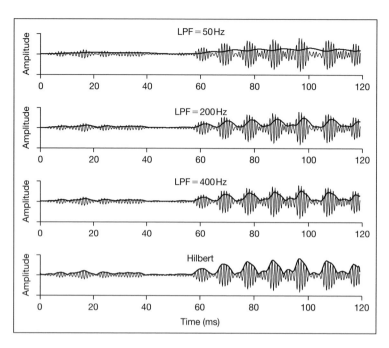

Fig. 7. Examples of envelope extraction based on full-wave rectification and low-pass filtering (top three panels) and the Hilbert transform (bottom panel). Envelopes are shown for three different envelope cutoff frequencies.

fine-structure waveform is a frequency-modulated signal (fig. 6) since the carrier frequency is not fixed but varies with time. Figure 6 shows an example of the decomposition of the time-domain waveform of the vowel /a/ into its envelope and fine-structure. It is clear from figure 6 that the Hilbert envelope contains periodicity information and therefore is not the same as the envelope defined by Rosen [40]. The Hilbert transform renders Rosen's [40] three-way partition of the temporal structure of speech into a two-way partition: the envelope, which also contains periodicity information, and the fine structure. This envelope/fine-structure decomposition of the signal (fig. 6) can be done independently for each channel. Figure 7 shows examples of envelopes extracted using the above two methods: the Hilbert transform and rectification followed by low-pass filtering. Of the two methods, the Hilbert transform produces more accurate estimates of the envelope. Use of higher envelope cutoff frequencies, however, yields envelopes close to those extracted by the Hilbert transform (fig. 7).

Current implant devices transmit envelope information, $a_i(t)$, and discard fine-structure information, $\cos[f_i(t)]$, as they implement only the analysis part of the vocoder and not the synthesis part (compare fig. 1 with fig. 3). Simulation studies [41–43] with normal-hearing listeners demonstrated the potential of including limited amounts of fine-structure information. It is not yet clear, however, how to incorporate fine-structure information in CIs in a way that they can perceive it [44].

Filter Spacing

For a given signal bandwidth (e.g. 0–8 kHz), there exist several ways of allocating the filters in the frequency domain. Some devices use a logarithmic spacing, while other devices use a linear spacing in the low frequencies ($<1,300$ Hz) and logarithmic spacing thereafter ($>1,300$ Hz). The effect of filter spacing on speech recognition, melody recognition and pitch perception has been investigated in a number of studies [45–48].

Fourakis et al. [47] advocated the placement of more filters in the F1/F2 region for better representation of the first two formants. They investigated the effect of filter spacing by modifying the electrode frequency boundary assignments of Nucleus 24 patients so as to include additional filters in the F1/F2 region. Small but significant improvements were noted on vowel recognition with an experimental MAP which included one additional electrode in the F2 region. No significant improvements were found on word recognition. The fixed number of frequency tables provided by the manufacturer, limited the investigators from assigning more electrodes in the F2/F3 region. The majority of the Nucleus-24 CI users tested preferred the experimental MAP over their everyday processor.

Similar findings were also found in our lab in patients newly implanted with the Clarion CII device fitted with 16 channels of stimulation. The effect of three different filter spacing, which included log, mel [49] and critical-band [50] spacing, was investigated on recognition of 11 vowels in /hVd/ format. Results (fig. 8) indicated that some subjects obtained a significant benefit with the critical-band spacing over the log spacing. Performance obtained with the mel frequency spacing was the lowest compared to the other two frequency spacing. This may be attributed to the number of frequency bands allotted in the F1 and F2 range. The mel frequency spacing had the smallest number (4) of bands allocated in the 0–1 kHz range, which is the F1 range for most vowels. In contrast, both the critical-band and the log spacing had 6 bands in the F1 range. In addition, the critical-band spacing had 7 bands in the 1–3 kHz range (F2 range), while the log spacing had 6.

The effect of filter spacing on pitch perception has been investigated in studies by Geurts and Wouters [51] and Laneau et al. [52], and will be discussed later. In brief, existing data support the idea that the number of filters allocated in the F1/F2 region can have a significant effect on performance, at least on vowel recognition tasks.

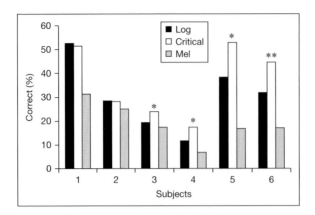

Fig. 8. Vowel recognition as a function of filter spacing (logarithmic, critical-band and mel) for 6 newly implanted Clarion CII users. The vowel test included vowels in /hVd/ format produced by 7 male speakers, 6 female speakers and 9 children. The stimuli were drawn from a set developed by Hillenbrand et al. [117]. Asterisks indicate significant differences (*p < 0.05, **p < 0.005) between the scores obtained with critical-band and log frequency spacing.

Spectral-Maxima Strategy

The spectral-maxima strategy implemented as the ACE (previously SPEAK) strategy on Cochlear Corporation devices [53] and as the 'n-of-m' strategy in other devices [54, 55], has antecedents in the channel-picking vocoders of the 1950s [56] as well as Haskins Laboratories' Pattern Playback speech synthesizer [57]. The principle underlying the use of this strategy is that speech can be well understood even when only the peaks in the short-term spectrum are transmitted. In the case of the Pattern Playback, only 4–6 of 50 harmonics needed to be transmitted to achieve highly intelligible speech – as long as the 'picked' harmonics defined the first two or three formants in the speech signal.

The spectral-maxima strategy is similar to the CIS strategy with the main difference being that the number of electrodes stimulated is smaller than the total number of analysis channels. In this strategy, the signal is processed through m band-pass filters from which only a subset n (n < m) of the envelope amplitudes are selected for stimulation. More specifically, the n maximum envelope amplitudes are selected for stimulation. The spectral-maxima strategy is sometimes called the 'n-of-m' strategy or peak-picking strategy and is available in both the Med-El and Nucleus-24 devices. In the Nucleus-24 device, out of a total of 20 envelope amplitudes, 10–12 maximum amplitudes are selected for stimulation in each cycle. The ACE (and SPEAK) strategy continuously estimates the outputs of the 20 filters and selects the ones with the largest amplitude. In the SPEAK strategy, the number of maxima selected varies from 5 to 10, depending on the spectral composition of the input signal, with an average number of six maxima. For broadband spectra, more maxima are selected and the stimulation rate is slowed down. For spectra with limited spectral content, fewer maxima are selected and the stimulation rate increases to provide more temporal information.

Several studies compared the performance of spectral-maxima and CIS strategies [15, 18, 58, 59]. CI simulation studies by Dorman et al. [59] indicated high performance with the spectral-maxima strategy even when a small number of maxima were selected in each cycle. A 3-of-20 processor (i.e. a processor that selected three maximum amplitudes out of 20 amplitudes in each cycle) achieved a 90% correct level of speech understanding for all stimulus material (sentences, vowels and consonants) presented in quiet. In contrast, it required 4, 6, and 8 channels of stimulation by CIS type processors to achieve similar levels of performance for sentences, consonants, and vowels, respectively. Hence, provided that there exist a large number of output analysis filters, only a small number of maxima need to be selected, an outcome consistent with the Pattern Playback studies. In noise (0 dB S/N), a minimum of 10 maxima needed to be selected for asymptotic performance on sentence recognition.

A study by Skinner et al. [15] compared the performance of Nucleus-24 implant patients fitted with the SPEAK, ACE and CIS strategies, after the patients used each strategy for a period of 4–6 weeks. Results indicated that the group mean score obtained with the ACE strategy on sentence recognition was significantly higher than the scores obtained with the SPEAK and CIS strategies. The SPEAK and ACE strategies are both spectral-maxima strategies selecting roughly the same number of envelope maxima (8–12) out of a total of 20 envelope outputs. The two strategies differ, however, in the stimulation rate. ACE's stimulation rate is significantly higher than SPEAK's and ranges from 900 to 1,800 pps while SPEAK's rate is fixed at 250 pps. The higher scores obtained with ACE can therefore be attributed to its higher stimulation rate.

Speech Coding Strategies Used in Commercial Devices

There are currently three CI processors in the United States approved by the Food and Drug Administration: the Nucleus 24, the Clarion and the Med-El processor. This section provides an overview of the signal processing strategies used in commercially available implant processors.

Advanced Bionics Corporation (Clarion CII/Auria Device)

The Advanced Bionics Corporation's (ABC's) implant has undergone a number of changes in the past decade. ABC's first generation implant (Clarion S-Series) included an electrode array with 8 contacts and supported a number of stimulation strategies including a simultaneous (analog-type) stimulation strategy [for review, see 60]. ABC's second generation device (termed Clarion CII) includes a 16-contact electrode array (HiFocus II) and supports simultaneous, partially simultaneous and nonsimultaneous stimulation strategies. Temporal bone studies have shown that the placement of the implanted Clarion's HiFocus II electrode array is extremely close to the modiolar wall [61].

The Clarion CII device supports a high-rate CIS strategy, which can be delivered either nonsimultaneously or partially simultaneously to 16 electrode contacts. Clarion's CIS strategy, called HiRes, differs from the traditional CIS strategy in the way it estimates the envelope. It uses half-wave rectification rather than full-wave rectification, and it does not use a low-pass filter. Instead, after the half-wave rectification operation, it averages the rectified amplitudes within each stimulation cycle. This averaging operation is in effect a low-pass filtering operation. The cutoff frequency of the low-pass filter depends on the number of samples to be averaged, i.e. it depends on the stimulation rate. The higher the stimulation rate (i.e. the smaller the number of samples to average), the higher the cutoff frequency.

In the HiRes strategy, the signal is first pre-emphasized and then band-pass filtered into 16 channels. The band-pass filters span the frequency range of 250–8,000 Hz and are logarithmically spaced. The filtered waveforms are half-wave rectified, averaged and logarithmically compressed to the patients' electrical dynamic range. The compressed envelopes are transmitted via RF to the implant decoder, where they are then modulated by trains of biphasic pulses for electrical stimulation. Comparisons between the conventional CIS strategy and the HiRes strategy were reported in studies by Filipo et al. [62] and Ostroff et al. [63].

The CII device utilizes a dual-action automatic gain control at the microphone input consisting of a slow-acting and a fast-acting stage. The slow-acting control has a compression threshold of 57 dB SPL with an attack time of 325 ms and a release time of 1,000 ms. The second control is fast acting and has a higher compression threshold of 65 dB SPL with an attack time of <0.6 ms and a release time of 8 ms.

The Clarion II device has 16 independent current sources that allow for simultaneous stimulation of two or more electrode contacts. When used in non-simultaneous mode of stimulation, HiRes operates at a stimulation rate of 2,800 pps/s using a pulse width of 11 μs/phase. The stimulation rate can be further increased by the use of partially simultaneous stimulation, whereby pairs of electrodes are stimulated simultaneously. To minimize potential channel inter-action, nonadjacent pairs of electrodes are typically selected (e.g. 1–8, 2–7, etc.). For 16 electrodes configured with paired pulses and a narrow pulse width, the stimulation rate can exceed 5,000 pps per channel. The combination of high rate stimulation and high cutoff frequency in the envelope detectors provides a fine temporal waveform representation of the signal at each channel. Some patients are able to utilize the fine temporal modulations present in the wave-form at such high stimulation rates [12, 62, 63].

The presence of multiple current sources allows for the implementation of virtual channel processing strategies, currently under investigation by ABC. By properly manipulating (or steering) the current delivered simultaneously to adjacent electrodes, it is possible to elicit pitches intermediate to the pitches elicited by each of the electrodes alone. These intermediate pitches may intro-duce intermediate 'virtual' channels of information. Different pitches can gen-erally be elicited by controlling the proportion of current delivered to each of the two electrodes [64]. Psychophysical studies have shown that simultaneous dual-electrode stimulation can produce as few as 2 and as many as 9 discrim-inable pitches between the pitches of single electrodes [65]. The motivation behind the virtual channel (also known as current-steering) idea is to produce intermediate pitches between electrodes in the hope of increasing the effective number of channels of information beyond the number of electrodes. The per-formance of the virtual channel strategy on music appreciation is currently being investigated by ABC. Anecdotal reports by some patients [e.g. 66] fitted with the virtual channel strategy were very encouraging.

Cochlear Corporation (Nucleus-24 ESPrit 3G/Freedom Device)

The Nucleus-24 device (CI24M) is equipped with an array of 22 banded intracochlear electrodes and two extracochlear electrodes, one being a plate electrode located on the implant package and the other a ball electrode located on a lead positioned under the temporalis muscle [67]. The electrode contacts of the Nucleus 24 Contour array are oriented toward the modiolus minimizing possible current spread away from the target spiral ganglion cells. The elec-trodes can be stimulated in a bipolar, monopolar or common ground configura-tion. The extracochlear electrodes are activated during monopolar stimulation and can be used individually or together. Biphasic stimulus pulses are generated with electrode shorting during the interstimulus gap (about 8 μs) to remove any residual charge.

The CI24M processor can be programmed with the ACE and CIS strate-gies [16]. Both strategies estimate the input signal spectrum using an FFT rather than a bank of band-pass filters. The filter bank is implemented using a 128-point Hanning Window and an FFT. Based on a sampling rate of 16 kHz, this provides an FFT channel spacing of 125 Hz and a low-pass filter cut-off frequency of 180 Hz. The FFT bins, which are linearly spaced in frequency, are used to produce n (12–22) filter bands, which are typically linearly spaced from 188 to 1,312 Hz and then logarithmically spaced up to 7,938 Hz. A total of n (n = 20) envelopes are estimated by summing the power of adjacent FFT bins within each of the n bands. In the ACE strategy, a subset of these envelope amplitudes is then selected in each stimulation time frame. More specifically, 8–12 maximum amplitudes are selected for stimulation. In the CIS strategy, a fixed number of amplitudes are used for stimulation based on processing the signal through a smaller number of bands (10–12). The remaining electrodes are inactivated. Electrodes corresponding to the selected bands are then stimulated in a tonotopic basal to apical order.

The stimulation rate can be chosen from a range of 250–2,400 pps per channel and is limited by a maximum rate of 14,400 pps across all channels. The stimulation rate can either be constant or jittered in time by a percentage of the average rate. When the jittered rate is programmed, the interstimulus gap (which is equal for all stimuli within one stimulation interval) is adjusted at every stimulation interval by a random amount. The resulting stimulation rate varies between consecutive stimulation intervals but has a fixed average rate.

For stimulation rates less than approximately 760 pps per channel, the filter bank analysis rate is set to equal to the stimulation rate. However, for higher stimulation rates, the analysis frequency is limited by the system to approximately 760 Hz and higher stimulation rates are obtained by repeating stimulus frames (stimuli in one stimulation interval) when necessary. For the 807 pps/channel rate, approximately 1 in every 17 or 18 stimulation frames is repeated. For the 1,615 pps/channel rate, approximately every stimulus frame is repeated.

The majority of the Nucleus users are fitted with the ACE strategy [67]. Comparisons between the performance of the ACE, SPEAK and CIS strategies on multiple speech recognition tasks can be found in Skinner et al. [15] and Parkinson et al. [67].

Med-El Corporation (COMBI-40+/Tempo+/PULSARci^{100} Device)

The Med-El CI processor is manufactured by Med-El Corporation, Austria [68]. The Med-El CI, also referred to as COMBI-40+, uses a very soft electrode carrier specially designed to facilitate deep electrode insertion into the cochlea [69]. Because of the capability of deep electrode insertion (approximately 31 mm), the electrodes are spaced 2.4 mm apart spanning a considerably larger distance (26.4 mm) in the cochlea than any other commercial CI. The motivation for using wider spacing between electrode contacts is to increase the number of perceivable channels and to minimize potential interaction between electrodes.

The implant processor can be programmed with either a high-rate CIS strategy or a high-rate spectral-maxima strategy. The Med-El processor has the capability of generating 18,180 pps for a high-rate implementation of the CIS strategy in the 12-channel COMBI-40+ implant. The amplitudes of the pulses are derived as follows. The signal is first pre-emphasized, and then applied to a bank of 12 (logarithmically spaced) band-pass filters. The envelopes of the band-pass filter outputs are extracted using the Hilbert transform [70]. Biphasic pulses, with amplitudes set to the mapped filter outputs, are delivered in an interleaved fashion to 12 monopolar electrodes at a default rate of of 1,515 pps per channel.

The latest Med-El device (PULSARci[100]) supports simultaneous stimulation of 12 electrodes. Higher (than the COMBI40+) stimulation rates are supported with aggregate rates up to 50,704 pps. For a 12-channel processor, rates as high as 4,225 pps/channel can be supported. Different stimulation techniques, including the use of triphasic pulses, are currently being explored by Med-El to reduce or minimize channel interaction associated with simultaneous stimulation.

Strategies Designed to Enhance F0 Information

The above strategies were originally designed to convey speech information but fall short on many respects in conveying adequate vocal pitch (F0) information. Speakers of tonal languages, such as Cantonese and Mandarin, make use of vocal pitch variations to convey lexical meaning. Several researchers have demonstrated that CI users fitted with current strategies have difficulty discriminating between several tonal contrasts [71, 72]. Also, CI users are not able to perceive several aspects of music including identification of familiar melodies and identification of musical instruments [73, 74]. Hence, strategies designed to improve coding of F0 information are critically important for better tonal language recognition and better music perception.

Pitch information can be conveyed in CIs via temporal and/or spectral (place) cues [52, 75–79]. Temporal cues are present in the envelope modulations of the band-pass filtered waveforms (fig. 7). Pitch can be elicited by varying the stimulation rate (periodicity) of a train of stimulus pulses presented on a single electrode, with high pitch percepts being elicited by high stimulation rates, and low pitch percepts being perceived by low stimulation rates. Once the stimulation rate increases beyond 300 Hz, however, CI users are no longer able to utilize such temporal cues to discriminate pitch [77]. Pitch may also be conveyed by electrode place of stimulation due to the tonotopic arrangement of the electrodes in the cochlea. Stimulation of apical electrodes elicits low pitch percepts while stimulation of basal electrodes elicits higher pitch percepts. Access to spectral cues is limited by the number of electrodes available (ranging from 12 to 22 in commercial devices), current spread causing channel interaction and possible pitch reversals due to suboptimal electrode placement.

A number of strategies have been proposed to enhance spectral (place) cues and/or temporal cues, and these strategies are described next.

Enhancing Spectral (Place) Cues

Two different strategies have been explored to improve place coding of F0 information. The first approach is based on the use of virtual channels via the means of dual-electrode (simultaneous) stimulation. By properly manipulating (or steering) the current delivered simultaneously to adjacent electrodes, it is possible to elicit pitches intermediate to the pitches elicited by each of the electrodes alone. These intermediate pitches may introduce intermediate 'virtual' channels of information. The virtual-channel approach is still in its infancy stages, and is currently being evaluated by several labs.

The second approach is based on modifying the shape of the filter response and/or the filter spacing. Such an approach was taken in three studies [48, 51, 52]. A new filter bank was proposed by Geurts and Wouters [51] based on a simple loudness model used in acoustic hearing. The filter was designed such that the loudness of a pure tone sweeping through the filter increased linearly with the frequency from the lower 3-dB cutoff frequency to the center frequency of each band, and decreased linearly from the center frequency to the upper boundary frequency. The resulting shape of the filters was triangular, with considerable overlap between adjacent filters. More filters were allocated in the low frequencies compared to a conventional filter-bank, which was based on log spacing. The new filter bank was tested on an F0 detection task. A 20-Hz low-pass filter was applied to the filter bank envelope signals to remove temporal cues. The new technique provided lower F0 detection thresholds for synthetic vowel stimuli compared to a conventional filter bank approach. However, when temporal cues to F0 were reintroduced, differences in detection thresholds between filter banks were reduced indicating that the temporal cues also provided some information about F0.

Kasturi and Loizou [48] proposed the use of semitone-based filter spacing for better music perception. Results with CI simulations indicated that the semitone filter spacing consistently yielded better performance than the conventional filter spacing. Nearly perfect melody recognition was achieved with only four channels of stimulation based on the semitone filter spacing. Subsequent studies with Clarion CII users indicated that some subjects performed significantly better with 6 channels based on semitone spacing than with 16 channels spaced logarithmically as used in their daily strategy.

Enhancing Temporal Cues

The strategies designed to enhance temporal cues can be divided into two main categories: those that explicitly code F0 information in the envelope and those that aim to increase the modulation depth of the filtered waveforms in the hope of making F0 cues perceptually more salient.

The idea of modulating the extracted envelope by explicit F0 information is not new and dates back to the original channel vocoder synthesizer (fig. 2), which was based on a source-filter excitation approach. In channel-vocoded speech, voiced segments of speech are generated by exciting the vocal tract by a periodic (glottal) pulse train consisting of pulses spaced 1/F0 s apart. Note that the F0 modulation idea was initially used in feature extraction strategies in the Nucleus device and later abandoned because of the inherent difficulty in extracting reliably F0 from the acoustic signal, particularly in noise. Jones et al. [80] investigated a strategy that provided F0 timing information on the most apical electrode. Results from several pitch perception tasks did not demonstrate any advantages with this approach.

Green et al. [5, 81, 82] adopted a similar approach to the enhancement of temporal pitch cues, based on the principle that F0 could be automatically extracted from voiced segments of the speech signal and used to appropriately modulate the envelopes. In the proposed strategy, amplitude envelopes were effectively split into two separate components. The first component contained slow-rate information of 32 Hz conveying the dynamic changes in the spectral envelope that are important for speech. The second component presented F0 information in the form of a simplified synthesized waveform. More specifically, F0-related modulation was presented in the form of a sawtooth waveform, on the assumption that 'such a "temporally sharpened" modulation envelope, with a rapid onset in each period, would lead to more consistent inter-pulse intervals in the neural firing pattern, and therefore to more salient temporal pitch cues' [5]. Implant users were required to label the direction of pitch movement of processed synthetic diphthong glides. Results indicated a significant advantage for the modified processing compared to standard CIS processing, demonstrating that the modified processing scheme was successful in enhancing the salience of temporal pitch cues. Subsequent studies by Green et al. [82], however, on tests of intonation perception and vowel perception indicated that the CI users performed worse with the F0-modified processing in vowel recognition compared to the conventional CIS strategy. The investigators concluded that while the modified processing enhanced pitch perception [5], it harmed the transmission of spectral information.

The above strategies assumed access to explicit F0 information. A number of strategies were proposed that did not rely on automatic extraction of F0 from the acoustic signal. These techniques focused on 'sharpening' the envelopes so as to make the F0 information more apparent or perceptually more salient. This was accomplished by increasing the modulation depth of the envelopes. Geurts and Wouters [83] proposed a simple modification to the estimation of the envelope. Two fourth-order low-pass filters were first employed with cutoff frequencies of 400 and 50 Hz. Note that the envelope output of the 400-Hz filter contained F0 modulations, but the envelope output of the 50-Hz filter did not. The modulation depth of the envelope was increased by subtracting an attenuated version of the 50-Hz (flat) log-compressed envelope from the 400-Hz log-compressed envelope. The resulting envelope was half-wave rectified (negative values set to zero), scaled and finally encoded for stimulation (note that the envelopes were already compressed to the patient's dynamic range prior to the subtraction operation). Despite the increase in modulation depth with the modified envelope processing, no significant differences in F0 discrimination of synthetic vowels were observed compared to the conventional CIS strategy [83]. Figure 9 shows examples of envelopes extracted with the above scheme and compared with envelopes extracted with conventional rectification and low-pass filtering (400 Hz).

The subtraction of the 400-Hz envelope amplitude from the 50-Hz envelope is equivalent to subtraction of the mean (dc component) of the rectified envelope, and constitutes a simple method for increasing envelope modulation depth. This idea was incorporated in one of the strategies proposed by Vandali et al. [6] to increase the modulation depth of the envelopes. The so-called, multi-channel envelope modulation (MEM) strategy utilized the envelope of the broadband signal (input acoustic signal prior to band-pass filtering), which inherently contains F0 periodicity information, to modulate the envelopes derived from the ACE filter bank. The envelope of the broadband signal was first estimated by full wave rectifying the broadband signal and then applying a 300-Hz, fourth-order low-pass filter. The modulation depth in the envelope signal was then expanded by applying an 80-Hz, second-order high-pass filter (HPF), which effectively increased the modulation depth of the envelope signal level by removing the mean (dc) component. Note that this step is equivalent to that of subtracting the mean of the rectified signal as done in the study by Geurts and

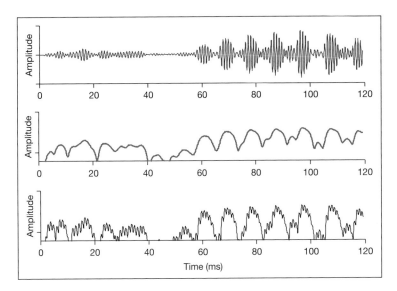

Fig. 9. Envelope output (bottom panel) obtained by the algorithm proposed by Geurts and Wouters [83] for enhancement of F0 cues. Top panel shows the filtered waveform of channel 6 (centered at 1 kHz) taken from the syllable /pa/ produced by a male speaker. Middle panel shows the corresponding envelope extracted using full-wave rectification and low-pass filtering (400 Hz), and subsequently log compressed to fit within a narrow electrical dynamic range. Bottom panel shows the envelope obtained by subtracting an attenuated version of the 50-Hz (flat) log-compressed envelope from the 400-Hz log-compressed envelope.

Wouters [83]. The low-pass filtered signal, obtained prior to the HPF stage, was scaled and added to the output of the HPF stage. The expanded envelope signal was then half-wave rectified, to remove any negative values, and scaled. Finally, the narrow-band envelope signals estimated by the ACE filter bank were low-pass filtered, using a 50-Hz, second-order low-pass filter, and then modulated by the normalized F0 envelope signal derived from the broadband signal. Figure 10 shows an example of the processed signal at different stages of the algorithm. As can be seen, the derived envelope has large modulation depth and the F0 periodicity is evident in the envelopes. Note also that the envelopes are temporally synchronized (across all electrodes) with the input (broadband) waveform.

The second strategy, termed Modulation Depth Enhancement (MDE) strategy, evaluated by Vandali et al. [6] provided explicit modulation expansion by decreasing the amplitude of the temporal minima of the envelope. Modulation depths smaller than a specified level were expanded using a third-order power function, and modulation depths above this level, but below an upper limit of 20 dB, were linearly expanded. The modulation depth expansion was implemented

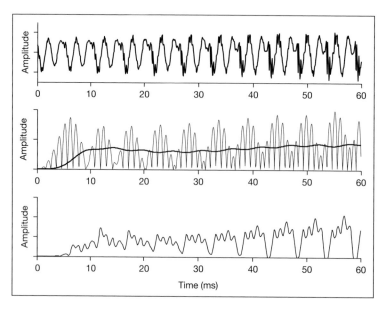

Fig. 10. Envelope outputs obtained at different stages of the MEM algorithm proposed by Vandali et al. [6] for enhancement of F0 cues. Top panel shows the input (broadband) signal taken from the vowel /i/ produced by a female speaker (F0 = 188 Hz). Middle panel shows the full-wave rectified signal of the filtered waveform of channel 3 (centered at 486 Hz). The 50-Hz envelope extracted using full-wave rectification and low-pass filtering is superimposed. Bottom panel shows the envelope output produced by the MEM algorithm. All waveforms are shown prior to compression.

by decreasing the amplitude of temporal minima in the signal while preserving the peak levels (a sliding time window, of 10-ms duration, was employed to track the peaks and minima). The modified envelope signals replaced those of the original envelope signals derived from the filter bank, and processing continued as per the normal ACE strategy. Comparison of the above strategies with the conventional ACE strategy indicated significantly higher scores with the MDE and MEM strategies on pitch ranking tasks. Comparison of the new strategies, however, on speech recognition tasks indicated no significant differences in scores with the conventional ACE strategy.

In brief, most of the above F0 enhancement strategies have been shown to improve pitch perception on tasks requiring discrimination of small pitch differences. Further work is needed, however, to investigate the efficacy of these F0 enhancement strategies on tonal language recognition and music perception tasks requiring perception of much finer pitch differences across a wide range of frequencies.

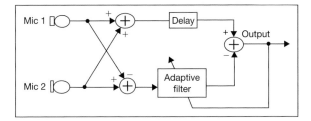

Fig. 11. Block diagram of the processing involved in the beamforming strategy based on two microphone inputs (Mic 1 and Mic 2).

Noise Reduction Strategies

Perhaps one of the most common complaints made by CI listeners is that their performance decreases rapidly in noisy environments. This is not surprising given the limited amount of spectral information that they receive with their CI [84, 85]. In noise, a larger number of channels are needed to understand speech [86, 87]. Increasing the number of effective channels of spectral information, however, has been one of the biggest challenges in CIs. For that reason, several researchers have focused on the development of noise reduction algorithms that either preprocess the noisy signal and feed the 'enhanced' signal to the input of the processor or somehow suppress the noise present in the envelope amplitudes.

Several noise reduction algorithms have been proposed for CI users. Some of those algorithms were based on the assumption that two or more microphones were available, while other algorithms assumed that the acoustic signal was picked up by a single microphone.

Multi-Microphone Methods

In some hearing aids and implant devices (e.g. Nucleus Freedom), a group of microphones with two or more entry ports are used with front and/or backward directivity. Some two-port microphones can reduce background noise simply by subtracting and delaying mechanically the input signals coming from each port of the diaphragm. Alternatively, the signals picked up by the two ports can be processed by an adaptive algorithm for better noise suppression.

The basis of the most sophisticated multi-microphone adaptive algorithms is the Griffiths-Jim beamforming algorithm [88] shown in figure 11. When the target signal comes from the front, the subtracter output at the bottom input (Mic 2) should contain primarily noise since the outputs from the two microphones will cancel each other. In contrast, the output of the adder in the top input (Mic 1) should contain a mixture of the noise and the signal of interest. These two outputs containing the noisy signal and reference noise signals, respectively, are fed as input to an adaptive filter shown to the right in figure 11. The LMS algorithm [89] is used to adapt the filter coefficients in such a way as to minimize the power of the output error (fig. 11). The error signal happens to be also the 'enhanced' signal that is fed to the input of a hearing aid or CI device. The above beamforming algorithm (fig. 11) has been found to work well in situations where there is only one noise source present and there is no reverberation.

Van Hoesel and Clark [90] tested an adaptive beamforming (ABF) technique, similar to that shown in Figure 11, with four Nucleus-22 users. The ABF method used signals from two microphones – one behind each ear – to reduce noise coming from 90° of the patients. The results of their study indicated that ABF with two microphones can bring substantial benefits to CI users in conditions for which reverberation is moderate and only one source is predominantly interfering with speech. The ABF strategy yielded significantly higher intelligibility scores compared to a strategy in which the two microphone signals were simply added together. Hamacher et al. [91] evaluated the performance of two ABF algorithms in different everyday-life noise conditions. The benefit of the two algorithms was evaluated in terms of the dB reduction in speech reception threshold. The mean benefit obtained using the beamforming algorithms for four CI users (wearing the Nucleus device) varied between 6.1 dB for meeting room conditions to 1.1 dB for cafeteria noise conditions.

Margo et al. [92] evaluated a two-microphone beamforming algorithm with 8 Nucleus users in a take-home trial for a period of 5–8 weeks. Subjective reports from the CI users indicated that the beamforming algorithm produced better sound quality and was preferred in noisy environments to their daily device. Wouters and van den Berghe [93] evaluated the performance of an ABF technique using a two-microphone array contained in a BTE hearing aid. The output of the noisy speech was preprocessed by the beamforming strategy and fed monaurally to the input of a LAURA CI processor. Speech was presented from the front and noise was presented from 90° of the patients. Results indicated significant improvement in speech intelligibility corresponding to an SNR improvement of about 10 dB.

In brief, multi-microphone-based methods can bring substantial benefits to speech intelligibility in noise particularly in situations where there is a single interferer present and there is no reverberation.

Single-Microphone Methods

In the above studies, it was assumed that two (or more) microphones were available, and in some cases that each microphone was placed behind each ear.

Adding, however, a second microphone contralateral to the implant is ergonomically difficult without requiring the CI users to wear headphones or a neck-loop, something that most patients would find cosmetically unappealing. Single-microphone noise reduction algorithms are therefore more desirable. These algorithms can be divided into two main categories: those that preprocess the noisy speech signal by a standard noise reduction algorithm and feed the 'enhanced' output to the input of the CI processor, and those that are embedded or integrated within the subject's CI coding strategy.

A number of preprocessing noise reduction strategies have been proposed for CIs, some of which were implemented on old CI processors that were based on feature extraction strategies. Hochberg et al. [94] used the INTEL noise reduction algorithm to preprocess speech and presented the processed speech to 10 Nucleus implant users fitted with the F0/F1/F2 and MPEAK feature extraction strategies [1]. Consonant-vowel-consonant words embedded in speech-shaped noise at S/N ratios in the range −10 to 25 dB were presented to the CI users. Significant improvements in performance were obtained at S/N ratios as low as 0 dB. The improvement in performance was attributed to more accurate formant extraction, as the INTEL algorithm reduced the errors caused by the feature extraction algorithm. This was quantified later in a study by Weiss [95] who demonstrated that fewer formant extraction errors were made when the signal was first preprocessed with the INTEL algorithm.

A few preprocessing algorithms were also evaluated using the latest implant processors. Yang and Fu [96] evaluated the performance of a spectral-subtractive algorithm using subjects wearing the Nucleus-22, Med-El and Clarion devices. Significant benefits in sentence recognition were observed for all subjects with the spectral-subtractive algorithm, particularly for speech embedded in speech-shaped noise.

Loizou et al. [97] evaluated a subspace noise reduction algorithm [98] which was based on the idea that the noisy speech vector can be projected onto 'signal' and 'noise' subspaces. The clean signal was estimated by retaining only the components in the signal subspace and nulling the components in the noise subspace. The performance of the subspace reduction algorithm was evaluated using 14 subjects wearing the Clarion device. Results indicated that the subspace algorithm produced significant improvements in sentence recognition scores compared to the subjects' daily strategy, at least in continuous (stationary) noise.

All the above methods, including the multi-microphone methods, were based on preprocessing the noisy signal and presenting the 'enhanced' signal to the CI users. The preprocessing approach has three main drawbacks, however: (1) preprocessing algorithms sometimes introduce unwanted distortion, e.g. musical noise [99], in the signal despite the fact that these algorithms improve the SNR, (2) preprocessing algorithms can be highly complex (power hungry) and do not work synergistically with existing CI strategies, and (3) there is no simple approach for optimizing the algorithm to individual users, and consequently we often do not know why some users benefit while others do not. Ideally, noise reduction algorithms should be easy to implement and be integrated into the existing coding strategies. Only a few algorithms [100, 101] were proposed along this direction.

Toledo et al. [100] proposed a simple envelope subtraction algorithm based on the principle that the clean (noise-free) envelope can be estimated by simply subtracting the noisy envelope from the noise envelope. This approach requires estimate of the noise envelope, which can be obtained using a noise estimation algorithm – an algorithm that continuously tracks the noise envelope even during speech activity. Results with four Clarion users indicated that some benefited with the envelope subtraction strategy. The lack of consistent improvement was attributed to inaccurate estimates of the noise envelope, which in turn might have produced speech distortion.

Loizou et al. [101] proposed the use of S-shaped compression functions in place of the conventional logarithmic compression functions for noise suppression. The motivation behind the use of S-shaped functions is to suppress the signal falling below the noise floor (and dominated by noise) while retaining the signal above the noise floor (and dominated by speech). This can be accomplished by the use of an expansive function for signal levels below the noise floor and a compressive function for signal levels above the noise floor (fig. 12). In a way, the expansive segment of the function serves as a signal attenuator, while the compressive segment serves as a signal amplifier. Key to the application of this S-shaped function is the choice of the knee point, which in the study by Loizou et al. [101] was set to the noise floor estimated using an algorithm. This knee point is not fixed, but adapted from cycle to cycle to the current estimate of the noise floor. Note that a similar input-output function is used in hearing aids [102], but with the knee point fixed at a specific input level (e.g. 50 dB SPL). In the study by Loizou et al. [101], a noise estimation algorithm [103] was used to track continuously the noise floor and adapt the knee point accordingly. The S-shaped function was evaluated with 7 Clarion CII users using IEEE sentences [104] embedded in +5 dB multi-talker babble. Results (fig. 13) showed significant improvements with the S-shaped compression compared to the log compression used in the subject's daily strategy.

Summary and Future Challenges

This paper provided an overview of the various speech processing strategies developed for CIs since the late 1990s. Many of those strategies, if not all,

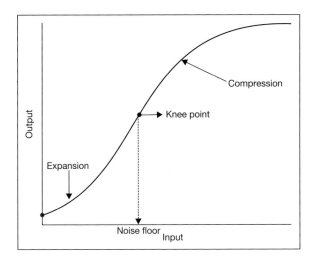

Fig. 12. The S-shaped input-output function.

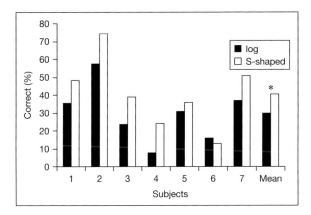

Fig. 13. Recognition (in terms of percent of words identified correctly) of sentences embedded in +5 dB multi-talker babble by 7 Clarion CII patients for two different input-output functions, logarithmic (as used in their daily strategy) and S-shaped (fig. 12). The S-shaped input-output function (fig. 12) was implemented using $y = A_1 x^{1.8} + A_2$ as the expansion function for signal levels below the knee point and $y = A_3 x^{-0.0001} + A_4$ as the compression function for signal levels above the knee point, where Ai are constants chosen to limit the acoustic dynamic range to the patient's electrical dynamic range. The differences in the mean scores were found to be statistically significant (*$p < 0.05$).

were variants of the Dudley's channel vocoder developed 60 years ago [2]. In fact, the latest attempts to design strategies to enhance F0 cues were similar to those used in the vocoder synthesizer (fig. 2). These strategies have been shown to improve pitch perception but have not yet been shown to improve music or tonal language perception. This paper also presented an overview of the signal processing strategies available in commercial processors. It also described work already in progress in our lab and elsewhere in developing noise suppression strategies based on multi-microphone and single-microphone inputs.

The overview presented here was by no means comprehensive. Several other strategies have been proposed but not described. These include the strategies designed to enhance onset cues [105–107], spectral contrast [101, 108] and to provide a closer mimicking of the function of the normal cochlea [109]. Such strategies are currently under evaluation.

Despite the success of the current strategies in improving speech understanding, there still remain several challenges ahead including (but not limited to) the following:

- development of strategies for better music perception,
- development of noise suppression strategies for improved speech recognition in noisy environments,
- development of strategies tailored to individual patients (such strategies will bridge the gap between the poorly-performing users and the 'star' users).

The development of such strategies will no doubt require a better understanding of: (a) the mechanisms used for complex pitch perception in electrically evoked hearing [51, 110]; (b) the acoustic cues used by CI users for understanding speech in noise [111] and the factors influencing CI users' ability to receive release of masking when listening to speech embedded in fluctuating maskers [112, 113]; (c) the factors influencing individual CI user's performance and the methods needed to assess the degree at which CI users are able to perceive temporal and/or spectral information. Such methods will help us design strategies that are tailored to individual CI user's perceptual capabilities.

Aside from the increased effort in the community to improve the design of speech coding strategies, there has also been effort to extend the capabilities of existing CI devices. Recent developments in CIs include the use of bilateral implants and combined acoustic and electric stimulation for subjects with residual hearing [for review, see 109]. Results with bilateral implant patients [114] and acoustic and electric stimulation patients [115] have shown great promise in improving speech understanding in noise. Bilateral implants have also improved the ability of CI users to localize sounds [114]. Further research is needed in developing strategies that use coordinated stimulation of the two implant processors (currently, operating independently of one another) for perhaps better preservation of interaural time delay cues.

In closing, it seems safe to expect further improvements in implant design and performance in the future, particularly regarding complex listening tasks such as listening to (and enjoying) Mozart's symphonies and conversing in crowded restaurants.

Acknowledgments

The writing of this paper was partially supported by grant No. R01 DC007527 from the National Institute of Deafness and Other Communication Disorders, NIH.

References

1   Loizou P: Mimicking the human ear: an overview of signal processing techniques for converting sound to electrical signals in cochlear implants. IEEE Signal Processing Mag 1998;15:101–130.
2   Dudley H: Remaking speech. J Acoust Soc Am 1939;11:1969–1977.
3   Schroeder M: Vocoders: analysis and synthesis of speech. Proc IEEE 1966;54:720–734.
4   Gold B, Rader C: The channel vocoder. IEEE Trans Audio Electroacoust 1967;15:148–161.
5   Green T, Faulkner A, Rosen S: Enhancing temporal cues to voice pitch in continuous interleaved sampling cochlear implants. J Acoust Soc Am 2004;116:2298–2310.
6   Vandali A, Sucher C, Tsang D, McKay C, Chew J, McDermott H: Pitch ranking ability of cochlear implant recipients: a comparison of sound-processing strategies. J Acoust Soc Am 2005;117: 3126–3138.
7   Shannon R, Zeng F-G, Kamath V, Wygonski J, Ekelid M: Speech recognition with primarily temporal cues. Science 1995;270:303–304.
8   Dorman M, Loizou P, Rainey R: Speech intelligibility as a function of the number of channels of stimulation for signal processors using sine-wave and noise-band outputs. J Acoust Soc Am 1997;102:2403–2411.
9   Eddington D: Speech discrimination in deaf subjects with cochlear implants. J Acoust Soc Am 1980;68:885–891.
10 Wilson CF, Lawson D, Wolford R, Eddington D, Rabinowitz W: Better speech recognition with cochlear implants. Nature 1991;352:236–238.
11 Wilson B, Lawson D, Zerbi M: Advances in coding strategies for cochlear implants. Adv Otolaryngol – Head Neck Surg 1995;9:105–129.
12 Loizou P, Poroy O, Dorman M: The effect of parametric variations of cochlear implant processors on speech understanding. J Acoust Soc Am 2000;108:790–802.
13 Brill S, Gstottner W, Helms J, Ilberg CV, Baumgartner W, Muller J, et al: Optimization of channel number and stimulation rate for the fast CIS strategy in the COMBI 40+. Am J Otol 1997;18: S104–S106.
14 Frijns J, Klop W, Bonnet R, Briare J: Optimizing the number of electrodes with high-rate stimulation of the Clarion CII cochlear implant. Acta Otolaryngol 2003;123:138–142.
15 Skinner M, Holden L, Whitford L, Plant K, Psarros C, Holden T: Speech recognition with the Nucleus 24 SPEAK, ACE and CIS speech coding strategies in newly implanted adults. Ear Hear 2002;23:207–223.
16 Vandali A, Whitford L, Plant K, Clark G: Speech perception as a function of electrical stimulation rate using the Nucleus 24 cochlear implant system. Ear Hear 2000;21:608–624.
17 Friesen L, Shannon R, Cruz R: Effects of stimulation rate on speech recognition with cochlear implants. Audiol Neurootol 2005;10:169–184.

18   Kim H, Shim Y, Chung M, Lee Y: Benefit of ACE compared to CIS and SPEAK coding strategies. Adv Otorhinolaryngol 2000;57:408–411.

19   Javel E: Acoustic and electrical encoding of temporal information; in Miller J, Spelman F (eds): Cochlear Implants: Models of the Electrically Stimulated Ear. NY, Springer-Verlag, 1990, pp 247–295.

20   Van den Honert C, Stypulkowski P: Physiological properties of the electrically stimulated auditory nerve II. Single fiber recordings. Hear Res 1984;14:225–243.

21   Rubinstein J, Wilson B, Finley C, Abbas P: Pseudospontaneous activity: stochastic independence of auditory nerve fibers with electrical stimulation. Hear Res 1999;127:108–118.

22   Litvak L, Delgutte B, Eddington D: Improved neural representation of vowels in electric stimulation using desynchronizing pulse trains. J Acoust Soc Am 2003;114:2099–2111.

23   Hong R, Rubinstein J: High-rate conditioning pulse trains in cochlear implants: dynamic range measures with sinusoidal stimuli. J Acoust Soc Am 2003;114:3327–3342.

24   Morse R, Evans E: Enhancement of vowel coding for cochlear implants by addition of noise. Nature 1996;2:928–932.

25   Zeng F-G, Fu Q, Morse R: Human hearing enhanced by noise. Brain Research 2001;869:251–255.

26   Boothroyd A, Erickson FN, Medwetsky L: The hearing aid input: a phonemic approach to assessing the spectral distribution of speech. Ear Hear 1994;6:432–442.

27   Zeng F-G, Grant G, Niparko J, Galvin J, Shannon R, Opie J, et al: Speech dynamic range and its effect on cochlear implant performance. J Acoust Soc Am 2002;111:377–386.

28   Eddington D, Dobelle W, Brachman D, Mladevosky M, Parkin J: Auditory prosthesis research using multiple intracochlear stimulation in man. Annals of Otology, Rhinology and Laryngology 1978;87(suppl 53):1–39.

29   Zeng F-G, Shannon R: Loudness balance between acoustic and electric stimulation. Hear Res 1992;60:231–235.

30   Fu Q-J, Shannon R: Effect of acoustic dynamic range on phoneme recognition in quiet and noise by cochlear implant users. J Acoust Soc Am 1999;106:L65–L70.

31   Fu Q-J, Shannon R: Effect of amplitude nonlinearity on phoneme recognition by cochlear implant users and normal-hearing listeners. J Acoust Soc Am 1998;104:2570–2577.

32   Fu Q-J, Shannon R: Phoneme recognition by cochlear implant users as a function of signal-to-noise ratio and nonlinear amplitude mapping. J Acoust Soc Am 1999;106:L18–L23.

33   Wilson B, Lawson D, Zerbi M, Wolford R: Speech Processors for Auditory Prostheses. NIH Project N01-DC-8-2105, Third Quarterly Progress Report 1999.

34   Zeng F-G, Galvin J: Amplitude mapping and phoneme recognition in cochlear implant listeners. Ear Hear 1999;20:60–74.

35   McKay CM, McDermott HJ, Clark GM: Pitch percepts associated with amplitude-modulated current pulse trains in cochlear implantees. J Acoust Soc Am 1994;96:2664–2673.

36   Wilson B, Zerbi M, Finley C, Lawson D, van Honert C: Speech Processors for Auditory Prostheses. NIH Project N01-DC-5-2103, Eighth Quarterly Progress Report 1997.

37   Drullman R: Temporal envelope and fine structure cues for speech intelligibility. J Acoust Soc Am 1995;97:585–592.

38   Lobo A, Toledo F, Loizou P: The effect of envelope cutoff frequency on consonant and melody recognition by CI listeners. J Acoust Soc Am 2002;112:2245.

39   Hartmann W. Signals, sounds and sensation. New York: Springer-Verlag, 1998.

40   Rosen S: Temporal information in speech: acoustic, auditory and linguistic aspects. Phil Trans R Soc Lond B Biol Sci 1992;336:367–373.

41   Zeng F-G, Nie K, Stickney G, Kong Y, Vongphoe M, Weit C, et al: Speech recognition with amplitude and frequency modulations. Proc Nat Acad Sciences 2005;102:2293–2298.

42   Smith ZM, Delgutte B, Oxenham AJ: Chimaeric sounds reveal dichotomies in auditory perception. Nature 2002;416:87–90.

43   Xu L, Pfingst B: Relative importance of temporal envelope and fine structure in lexical-tone perception. J Acoust Soc Am 2003;114:3204–3207.

44   Wilson B, Sun X, Schatzer R, Wolford R: Representation of fine structure or fine frequency information with cochlear implants. Int Congr Ser 2004;1273:3–6.

45 Skinner M, Holden L, Holden T: Effect of frequency boundary assignment on speech recognition with the SPEAK speech-coding strategy. Ann Otol Rhinol Laryngol 1995;104(suppl 166): 307–311.

46 Fu Q-J, Shannon R: Frequency mapping in cochlear implants. Ear Hear 2002;23:339–348.

47 Fourakis M, Hawks J, Holden L, Skinner M, Holden T: Effect of frequency boundary assignment on vowel recognition with the Nucleus 24 ACE speech coding strategy. J Am Acad Audiol 2004;15:281–289.

48 Kasturi K, Loizou P: Effect of filter spacing and correct tonotopic representation on melody recognition: implications for cochlear implants. Proceedings of ARO, New Orleans, LA 2005.

49 Fant G: Speech Sounds and Features. Boston, MIT Press, 1973.

50 Zwicker E, Fastl H: Psychoacoustics, Facts and Models. Berlin, Springer Verlag, 1990.

51 Geurts L Wouters J: Better place-coding of the fundamental frequency in cochlear implants. J Acoust Soc Am 2004;115:844–852.

52 Laneau J, Moonen M, Wouters J: Relative contributions of temporal and place pitch cues to fundamental frequency discrimination in cochlear implantees. J Acoust Soc Am 2004;106: 3606–3619.

53 McDermott H, McKay C, Vandali A: A new portable sound processor for the University of Melbourne/Nucleus Limited multielectrode cochlear implant. J Acoust Soc Am 1992;91: 3367–3371.

54 Wilson B, Finley C, Farmer J, Lawson D, Weber B, Wolford R, et al: Comparative studies of speech processing strategies for cochlear implants. Laryngoscope 1998;98:1069–1077.

55 Wilson B, Finley C, Farmer J, Lawson D, Weber B, Wolford R, et al: Comparative studies of speech processing strategies for cochlear implants. Laryngoscope 1988;1069–1077.

56 Peterson G, Cooper F: Peakpicker: a bandwidth compression device. J Acoust Soc Am 1957; 29:777A.

57 Cooper F, Liberman A, Borst J: Preliminary studies of speech produced by a pattern playback. J Acoust Soc Am 1950;22:678.

58 Kiefer J, Muller J: Speech understanding in quiet and in noise with the CIS speech coding strategy (Med-El Combi-40) compared to the multi-peak and SPEAK strategies. ORL J Otorhinolaryngol Relat Spec 1996;58:127–135.

59 Dorman M, Loizou P, Spahr T, Maloff E: A comparison of the speech understanding provided by acoustic models of fixed-channel and channel-picking signal processors for cochlear implants. J Speech Lang Hear Res 2002;45:783–788.

60 Loizou P, Stickney G, Mishra L, Assmann P: Comparison of speech processing strategies used in the Clarion implant processor. Ear Hear 2003;24:12–19.

61 Balkany T, Esharaghi A, Yang N: Modioloar proximity of three perimodiolar cochlear implant electrodes. Acta Otolaryngol 2002;122:363–369.

62 Filipo M, Mancini P, Ballantyne D, Bosco E, D'Elia C: Short-term study of the effect of speech coding strategy on the auditory performance of pre- and post-lingually deafened adults implanted with the Clarion CII. Acta Otolaryngol 2004;124:368–370.

63 Ostroff J, David E, Shipp D, Chen J, Nedzelski J: Evaluation of the high-resolution coding strategy for the Clarion CII cochlear implant system. J Otolaryngol 2003;32:81–86.

64 Wilson B, Zerbi M, Lawson D: Speech processors for auditory prostheses. NIH Contract N01-DC-2–2401, 3rd Quarterly Progress Report, February 1– April 30 1993.

65 Donaldson G, Kreft H, Litvak L: Place-pitch discrimination of single- versus dual-electrode stimuli by cochlear implant users. J Acoust Soc Am 2005;118:623–626.

66 Chorost M: My bionic quest for Bolero. Wired Magazine 2005;11:144–159.

67 Parkinson A, Arcaroli J, Staller S, Arndt P, Cosgriff A, Ebinger K: The Nucleus 24 Contour cochlear implant system: adult clinical trial results,'. Ear Hear 2002;23:41S-48S.

68 Bassim M, Buss E, Clark M, Kolln K, Pillsbury C, Pillsbury H, et al: MED-EL Combi-40+ cochlear implantation in adults. Laryngoscope 2005;115:1568–1573.

69 Kos M, Boex C, sigrist A, Guyot J, Pelizzone M: Measurements of electrode position inside the cochlea for different cochlear implant systems. Acta Otolaryngol 2005;125:474–480.

70 Zierhofer C: Cochlear implant system. United States Patent 5,983,139. 1999.

71   Barry J, Blamey P, Martin L, Lee K, Tang T, Ming Y, et al: Tone discrimination in Cantonese-speaking children using a cochlear implant. Clin Linguist Phon 2002;6:99.

72   Fu Q-J, Zeng F-G, Shannon R, Soli S: Importance of tonal envelope cues in Chinese speech recognition. J Acoust Soc Am 1998;104:505–510.

73   Gfeller K, Lansing CR: Melodic, rhythmic, and timbral perception of adult cochlear implant users. J Speech Hear Res 1991;34:916–920.

74   Gfeller K, Woodworth G, Robin DA, Witt S, Knutson JF: Perception of rhythmic and sequential pitch patterns by normally hearing adults and adult cochlear implant users. Ear Hear 1997;18: 252–260.

75   Tong Y, Clark G: Absolute identification of electric pulse rates and electrode positions by cochlear implant patients. J Acoust Soc Am 1985;77:1881–1888.

76   Townshend B, Cotter N, van Compernolle D, White RL: Pitch perception by cochlear implantees. J Acoust Soc Am 1987;82:106–115.

77   Zeng F-G: Temporal pitch in electric hearing. Hear Res 2002;174:101–106.

78   Carlyon R, Wieringen A, Long C, Deeks J, Wouters J: Temporal pitch mechanisms in acoustic and electric hearing. J Acoust Soc Am 2002;112:621–623.

79   Laneau J, Wouters J: Multi-channel place pitch sensitivity in cochlear implant recipients. J Assoc Res Otorlaryngol 2004;5:285–294.

80   Jones P, McDermott H, Seligman, Millar J: Coding of voice source information in the Nucleus cochlear implant system. Ann Otol Rhinol Laryngol 1995;104:363–365.

81   Green T, Faulkner A, Rosen S: Spectral and temporal cues to pitch in noise-excited vocoder simulations of continuous interleaved sampling cochlear implants. J Acoust Soc Am 2002;112:2155–2164.

82   Green T, Faulkner A, Rosen S, Macherey O: Enhancement of temporal periodicity cues in cochlear implants: effects on prosodic perception and vowel identification. J Acoust Soc Am 2005;118: 375–385.

83   Geurts L, Wouters J: Coding of the fundamental frequency in CIS processors for cochlear implants. J Acoust Soc Am 2001;109:713–726.

84   Fishman K, Shannon R, Slattery W: Speech recognition as a function of the number of electrodes used in the SPEAK cochlear implant processor. J Speech Hear Res 1997;40:1201–1215.

85   Friesen L, Shannon R, Baskent D, Wang X: Speech recognition in noise as a function of the number of spectral channels: comparison of acoustic hearing and cochlear implants. J Acoust Soc Am 2001;110:1150–1163.

86   Fu Q-J, Shannon R, Wang X: Effects of noise and spectral resolution on vowel and consonant recognition: acoustic and electric hearing. J Acoust Soc Am 1998;104:3586–3596.

87   Dorman M, Loizou P, Fitzke J, Tu Z: The recognition of sentences in noise by normal-hearing listeners using simulations of cochlear-implant signal processors with 6–20 channels. J Acoust Soc Am 1998;104:3583–3585.

88   Griffiths L, Jim C: An alternative approach to linearly contrasted adaptive beamforming. IEEE Trans Antennas Propagation 1982;30:27–34.

89   Widrow B, Stearns S: Adaptive Signal Processing. Englewood Cliffs, NJ, Prentice Hall, 1985.

90   Van Hoesel R, Clark G: Evaluation of a portable two-microphone adaptive beamforming speech processor with cochlear implant patients. J Acoust Soc Am 1995;97:2498–2503.

91   Hamacher V, Doering W, Mauer G, Fleischmann H, Hennecke J: Evaluation of noise reduction systems for cochlear implant users in different acoustic environments. Am J Otol 1997;18:S46-S49.

92   Margo V, Terry M, Schweitzer C, Shallop J: Results of take-home trial for a non-linear beam-former as a noise reduction strategy for cochlear implants. J Acoust Soc Am 1995;98:2984.

93   Wouters J, van den Berghe J: Speech recognition in noise for cochlear implantees with a two-microphone monaural adaptive noise reduction system. Ear Hear 2001;22:420–430.

94   Hochberg I, Boorthroyd A, Weiss M, Hellman S: Effects of noise and noise suppression on speech perception by cochlear implant users. Ear Hear 1992;13:263–271.

95   Weiss M: Effects of noise and noise reduction processing on the operation of the Nucleus-22 cochlear implant processor. J Rehab Res Dev 1993;30:117–128.

96   Yang L, Fu Q: Spectral subtraction-based speech enhancement for cochlear implant patients in background noise. J Acoust Soc Am 2005;117:1001–1004.

Loizou

97 Loizou P, Lobo A, Hu Y: Subspace algorithms for noise reduction in cochlear implants. J Acoust Soc Am 2005;118:2791–2793.

98 Hu Y, Loizou P: A generalized subspace approach for enhancing speech corrupted by colored noise. IEEE Trans on Speech and Audio Processing 2003;11:334–341.

99 Berouti M, Schwartz R, Makhoul J: Enhancement of speech corrupted by acoustic noise. Proc IEEE Int Conf Acoust, Speech, Signal Process 1979;208–211.

100 Toledo F, Loizou P, Lobo A: Subspace and envelope subtraction algorithms for noise reduction in cochlear implants. Conf of IEEE Engineering in Medicine and Biology Society 2003;3:17–21.

101 Loizou P, Kasturi K, Turicchia L, Sarpeshkar R, Dorman M, Spahr T: Evaluation of the companding and other strategies for noise reduction in cochlear implants. Abstr of 2005 Conference on Implantable Auditory Prostheses 2005.

102 Dillon H: Hearing Aids. NY, Thieme, 2001.

103 Rangachari S, Loizou P: A noise estimation algorithm for highly non-stationary environments. Speech Commun 2006;28:220–231.

104 IEEE Subcommittee: IEEE Recommended Practice for Speech Quality Measurements. IEEE Trans Audio and Electroacoustics 1969;17:225–246.

105 Geurts L, Wouters J: Enhancing the speech envelope of CIS processors for cochlear implants. J Acoust Soc Am 1999;105:2476–2484.

106 Vandali A: Emphasis of short-duration acoustic speech cues for cochlear implant users. J Acoust Soc Am 2001;109:2049–2061.

107 Holden L, Vandali A, Skinner M, Fourakis M, Holden T: Speech recognition with the ACE and transient emphasis spectral maxima strategies in Nucleus 24 recipients. J Speech Lang Hear Res 2005;48:681–701.

108 Turicchia L, Sarpeshkar R: A bio-inspired companding strategy for spectral enhancement. IEEE Transactions on Speech and Audio Processing 2005;13:243–253.

109 Wilson B, Lawson D, Muller J, Tyler R, Kiefer J: Cochlear implants: some likely next steps. Annu Rev Biomed Eng 2003;5:207–249.

110 McDermott H, McKay CM: Musical pitch perception with electrical stimulation of the cochlea. J Acoust Soc Am 1997;101:1622–1631.

111 Munson B, Nelson P: Phonetic identification in quiet and in noise by listeners with cochlear implants. J Acoust Soc Am 2005;118:2607–2617.

112 Qin M, Oxenham A: Effects of simulated cochlear-implant processing on speech reception in fluctuating maskers. J Acoust Soc Am 2003;114:446–454.

113 Stickney G, Zeng F-G, Litovsky R, Assmann P: Cochlear implant speech recognition with speech maskers. J Acoust Soc Am 2004;116:1081–1091.

114 Van Hoesel R, Tyler R: Speech perception, localization, and lateralization with bilateral cochlear implants. J Acoust Soc Am 2003;113:1617–1630.

115 Kiefer J, Tillein J, von Ilberg C, Pfennigdorff T, Strurzebecher E: Fundamental aspects and first results of the clinical application of combined electric and acoustic stimulation of the auditory system. Cochlear Implants – An update 2002;569–576.

116 Hartmann WM, Johnson D: Stream segregation and peripheral channeling. Music Percept 1991;9:155–184.

117 Hillenbrand J, Getty L, Clark M, Wheeler K: Acoustic characteristics of American English vowels. J Acoust Soc Am 1995;97:3099–3111.

Philipos C. Loizou, PhD
Department of Electrical Engineering
Jonsson School of Engineering and Computer Science
University of Texas at Dallas, PO Box 830688
Richardson, TX 75083–0688 (USA)
Tel. +1 972 883 4617, Fax +1 972 883 2710, E-Mail loizou@utdallas.edu

Møller AR (ed): Cochlear and Brainstem Implants.
Adv Otorhinolaryngol. Basel, Karger, 2006, vol 64, pp 144–153

·······················

Auditory Brainstem Implants: Surgical Aspects

Jose N. Fayad[a,b], *Steven R. Otto*[b], *Derald E. Brackmann*[a,b]

[a]House Clinic, [b]House Ear Institute, Los Angeles, Calif., USA

Abstract

Patients with neurofibromatosis type 2 often develop bilateral life-threatening vestibular schwannoma necessitating tumor removal, which results in deafness. We developed the auditory brainstem implant (ABI) in order to be able to electrically stimulate the cochlear nucleus complex in patients with bilateral cochlear nerve injury from bilateral schwannoma. After tumor removal, the electrode array of the ABI is inserted into the lateral recess of the fourth ventricle and placed over the surface of the ventral and dorsal cochlear nuclei. The ABI is designed to stimulate auditory neural structures within the cochlear nucleus in order to convey salient cues about the frequency, amplitude, and temporal characteristics of sounds. To date, more than 200 patients have received an ABI device at our institution. Recently, penetrating ABIs were introduced, and preliminary results of penetrating ABIs are discussed in this paper. The surgical anatomy of the nucleus and surgical placement of the ABI in patients with neurofibromatosis type 2 are described, and surgical considerations in this group of challenging patients are detailed.

Patients with neurofibromatosis type 2 (NF2) usually have bilateral vestibular schwannoma necessitating tumor removal, which often results in deafness. Cochlear implants, which electrically activate neural structures within the cochlea, are not an option for patients with NF2 because of their loss of integrity of the auditory nerve. We developed the auditory brainstem implant (ABI) in order to provide hearing for patients with NF2 whose auditory nerve had been destroyed. Drs. William House and William Hitselberger first used the ABI to stimulate the cochlear nucleus electrically in such a patient in 1979 [1–3]. The electrode array of the ABI is introduced into the lateral recess of the fourth ventricle and placed over the area of the ventral and dorsal cochlear nuclei after tumor removal. The ABI is similar in design and function to multichannel cochlear implants except for differences in the design of the stimulating electrode arrays [4–6]. The programming of ABI devices also differs in several important aspects from cochlear implant programming.

Multichannel cochlear implants and ABIs were developed to capitalize on the frequency tuning of neurons in the human cochlea and cochlear nucleus complex, respectively. In multichannel cochlear implants, the electrode is placed into the cochlea. Consistent placement of the electrode carrier and its depth of insertion are assured in normal cochleas. However in ABI recipients, anatomical landmarks that are used in electrode array placement may be altered or obscured from tumors making electrode array placement more challenging. This paper describes the surgical anatomy of the cochlear nucleus complex and our experience and results with ABIs in individuals with NF2. We also discuss the use of ABIs in patients with other kinds of auditory nerve pathologies.

Patient Selection

With two exceptions, only patients with NF2 and bilateral acoustic schwannoma have received the ABI at the House Clinic. In the NF2 patients, the goal is to restore some auditory function in order for these individuals to continue to be a part of the hearing world and to improve their quality of life. The ABI is placed during removal of their first tumor even if they have hearing on the other side, which is usually the case. This approach allows patients to become familiar with the use of the device and prepares them for the loss of hearing on the other side when they will be deaf in both ears [7–9].

Other possible indications for ABIs include bilateral transverse skull fractures with avulsion of both cochlear nerves. More recently, in Europe, the indications for the ABI have included cochlear nerve aplasia and severe cochlear malformations in children, and complete ossification of the cochlea or cochlear nerve disruption due to cochlear trauma in adults [10–12]. These indications are discussed in the paper by Colletti [this vol, pp 167–185].

Surgical Technique and Anatomy of the Cochlear Nucleus

The cochlear nucleus complex (dorsal and ventral cochlear nuclei) is part of the floor of the lateral recess of the fourth ventricle [13, 14]. The target for the placement of the electrode array is partially obscured by the cerebellar peduncles. A surface electrode introduced in the lateral recess crossing the tinea choroidea will stimulate viable cells in the cochlear nuclei.

At the House Clinic we have exclusively used the translabyrinthine approach for placement of the ABI. In the past, an italic S type of incision was used as for cochlear implants. This incision extended above the pinna for 4 cm. More

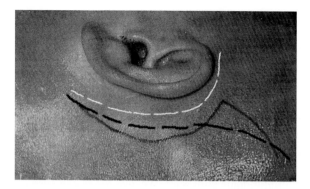

Fig. 1. C-shaped incision currently used for placement of an ABI (white line); previously used incisions are also marked in black and gray.

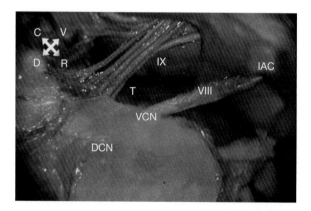

Fig. 2. Anatomy of the cochlear nuclei: anatomical preparation (left side) showing the internal auditory canal (IAC), cranial nerves VIII and IX converging towards the entrance of the lateral recess (foramen of Luschka) where the tinea (T) is. The location of ventral (VCN) and dorsal (DCN) cochlear nuclei is shown. C = Caudal; D = dorsal; R = rostral; V = ventral.

recently, we started using a C-shaped incision that extends just 1–1.5 cm above the pinna (fig. 1). It allows the placement of the internal receiver and magnet under the scalp. It is important that the incision does not directly cross the area where the receiver/stimulator is to be placed.

The translabyrinthine approach provides direct access to the cochlear nuclei. The jugular bulb is skeletonized to provide the widest access to this area. Anatomical landmarks used for placement of the implant include the stump of the eighth nerve, the glossopharyngeal nerve, the facial nerve and the tinea choroidea as well as the entrance to the lateral recess (foramen of Luschka) where all of these structures converge (figs. 2–4). The neurosurgeon in our team

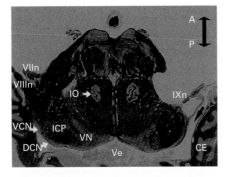

Fig. 3. Histological section showing the area of the lateral recess of the fourth ventricle (Ve), cranial nerves VII (VIIn), VIII (VIIIn), IX (IXn), and the relationship between ventral cochlear nucleus (VCN), dorsal cochlear nucleus (DCN), inferior cerebellar peduncle (ICP), and the vestibular nuclei (VN). The cerebellum (CE) and the inferior olive (IO) are also shown. A = Anterior; P = posterior.

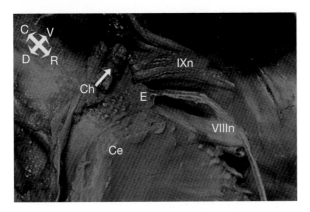

Fig. 4. View of the site of implantation on a cadaveric preparation. The electrode (E) is seen in the lateral recess over the area of the cochlear nucleus; the foramen of Luschka is outlined by the VIII (VIIIn) and IX (IXn) cranial nerves; the cerebellar peduncles (Ce) form the superior limit; the choroid plexus (Ch) usually protrudes from the lateral recess. C = Caudal; D = dorsal; R = rostral; V = ventral.

notes that the two features that he uses in identifying the foramen of Luschka are its relationship to the ninth cranial nerve and the position of the jugular bulb. In the surgical setting, where there is almost always distortion of the brain stem from the tumor, the foramen of Luschka is located superior to the ninth nerve. The ninth nerve is generally in a fixed anatomic position leading to foramen of Luschka in almost every case. The jugular bulb is important because its position may vary. Indeed, with a contracted mastoid and a high jugular bulb, the exposure may be more difficult although it should not be an impediment to placement of the ABI electrode array. The key is to have good exposure of the jugular bulb, which will augment the exposure of the foramen of Luschka.

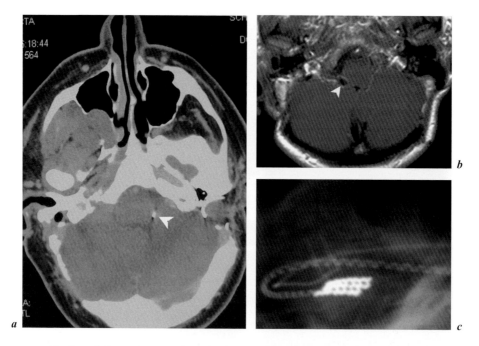

Fig. 5. *a* CT scan showing signal from (L) electrode (arrow). *b* MRI scan showing signal from (R) electrode (arrow). *c* X-ray showing ABI penetrating and surface electrodes.

The ventral cochlear nucleus is the main target for placement of the ABI. The correct placement is confirmed using electrophysiological recordings. Electrically evoked auditory brainstem responses elicited by stimulation of the nucleus are recorded from electrodes placed on the scalp, and the position of the ABI electrode is optimized using information derived from these recordings [15; see also Nevison, this vol, pp 154–166]. In addition to facial nerve monitoring, the lower cranial nerves are also monitored to detect stimulation of these nerves by the implant that may cause nonauditory sensations. Once the implant is placed in its optimal position, Teflon felt is used to secure the electrode array in the lateral recess of the fourth ventricle (fig. 5). The internal receiver is fixed to the skull in a posterosuperior position to the mastoid defect; a seat is created in the bone to lower the profile of the internal receiver/stimulator, which is stabilized using nonresorbable sutures to the skull. Others have used the retrosigmoid approach to implant the cochlear nucleus complex with similar results [12].

Similar technique is used to implant penetrating ABIs (PABI). After positioning of the penetrating part of the electrode array in the ventral portion of the

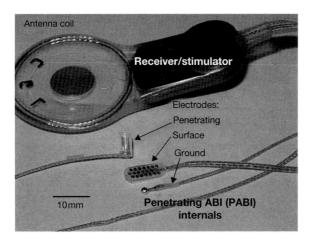

Fig. 6. The device: surface and penetrating electrodes side by side, also showing the ground (reference) electrode.

nucleus, the surface electrodes, which are part of the PABI, are placed in a way similar to a regular ABI.

Implantation is easier when the landmarks are preserved and the surface anatomy is normal as is the case in the newest indications for the ABI, i.e. cochlear nerve aplasia and severe cochlear malformations in children, and complete ossification of the cochlea in adults [10].

Device

The currently used surface ABI electrode array consists of 21 electrodes that are embedded in a silicone carrier that is fixed to a fabric mesh and connected to an implantable internal receiver/stimulator. The investigational PABI consists of two arrays, a 12-electrode surface array plus a 10-electrode array with needle microelectrodes (fig. 6). The external equipment for both devices consists of a transmitter coil held in place by magnetic tape placed on the scalp over the receiver/stimulator coil and connected to a sound processor, which contains the battery. This part of ABIs is similar to that of cochlear implants. However, for NF2 and other patients needing serial follow-up MRI scans, the internal magnet like found in cochlear implants is removed. Scans can be obtained as long as the external magnet/magnetic tape is removed because the implanted hardware is nonferromagnetic [16].

Both cochlear and ABIs have digital processors that operate on the signals from a microphone that is worn close to the ear [Loizou, this vol, pp 109–143].

The sound-processing unit (speech processor) requires appropriate programming and must be fitted to individual users. Programming speech processors involves psychophysical assessment of electrically induced auditory (and nonauditory) percepts including threshold, comfort level, and pitch.

In multichannel auditory implants, different sites of stimulation can generate different pitch perception for the wearer. Changes in the frequency spectrum of sound can therefore be coded by appropriate changes in the patterns of electrode activation. Cochlear implants can usually employ a relatively standard pattern of neural stimulation, because of the homogeneous tuning of neurons in the cochlea. ABI recipients, however, have variations in brainstem anatomy, electrode array placement, and tumor effects that require the use of more individualized stimulus patterns to code frequency cues, and manage any nonauditory sensations. Special techniques and additional time are usually required to program ABI sound processors appropriately.

Initial stimulation is carried out 1–2 months after the implantation. Nonauditory sensations are reduced or eliminated by selecting the configuration of the electrodes to be activated and the electrical parameters of stimulation (particularly pulse duration and reference electrode). Nonauditory sensations have included dizziness, sensation of vibration in the eye, throat sensations, and ipsilateral tingling sensations in the head or body.

The first 25 patients implanted with the ABI prior to 1992 at the House Ear Institute (HEI) received a single-channel system [4]. Since 1992, the Nucleus multichannel ABI device (Cochlear Corporation, Englewood, Colo., USA) has been used, which has resulted in improved performance [7]. This type of implant completed clinical trials and received final approval for commercial release from the U.S. Food and Drug Administration on October 20, 2000.

The PABI has two arrays (a surface and a penetrating array), and the processor allows three different programming modes to be used: surface electrodes only, penetrating electrodes only, or a combination of electrodes from both arrays. Performance is assessed with each of these configurations adding to the time necessary to manage these research patients.

Results

Many articles have been published detailing results from using ABIs. To date, more than 200 patients have been implanted using this device at HEI, and more than 500 recipients worldwide. The safety of this device has been comparable to the safety of cochlear implants. At our institution, only 2 patients (early users of the 'single-channel' ABI) had to be explanted due to infection.

Eighty percent of the patients use their ABI regularly, and approximately 90% have received auditory sensations from their ABIs. Approximately 16% of patients have achieved limited open-set speech discrimination (at least 20% correct in sound only on the CUNY Sentences Test) [4, 5, 7, 8; see also the paper by Colletti, this vol, pp 167–185]. A few ABI recipients have scored in the vicinity of 50% or better in sound only on this test. The majority of the patients recognize some environmental sounds; and speech understanding ability is enhanced an average of 30% when ABI sound is added to lip-reading cues. This enhancement has been as high as 70% improvement for some patients.

Results Using the Penetrating Electrode

The PABI was developed at HEI and Huntington Medical Research Institute (Pasadena, Calif., USA) in collaboration with the manufacturer, Cochlear Corporation. It was developed in an effort to improve the precision of stimulation of brainstem auditory neurons. The PABI is in the clinical trials phase under auspices of the US Food and Drug Administration. It was thought that microstimulation with needle electrodes would provide activation of smaller populations of tonotopic groups of neurons at lower current levels and with a range of pitch percepts.

Three PABI recipients implanted during phase I at HEI have been extensively tested over the past 2 years. The patients use their PABI devices daily, with benefit. The effects of each array, or a combination of electrodes from both arrays, are studied in each patient. Their performance has been stable, and speech perception as measured on CUNY Sentences is improved an average of 30% when using sound and lip-reading together (as compared to the lip-reading only condition). The patients have performed best on this test when using a speech processor program that combines surface with penetrating electrodes. Penetrating electrodes have lower thresholds for auditory sensations than surface electrodes. Some electrodes reach the charge limit while only yielding a sound sensation that is soft to moderately loud. An increase in the stimulating area of the surface electrodes and a slight increase in allowable charge may improve the usability of these electrodes, and these upgrades have been implemented in the second generation PABI. The recipients of the PABI report a wide range of pitch sensations on both penetrating and surface electrodes, which we believe is a factor that enhances speech perception performance. The study will continue with implantation of up to 10 patients with the second generation PABI.

Conclusion

The ABI electrode array is introduced using a translabyrinthine approach to the lateral recess of the fourth ventricle and placed over the surface of the ventral and dorsal cochlear nuclei after vestibular schwannoma removal. More than 200 patients have been implanted using the ABI at HEI, more than 500 worldwide. The safety of the stimulation of the cochlear nuclei using this device has been established. Most patients perceive useful auditory sensations and improve their communication abilities over lip-reading only. A smaller number achieve substantial speech discrimination using only ABI sound. The majority of ABI recipients typically use the device regularly and find that it improves their quality of life.

References

1   Edgerton BJ, House WF, Hitselberger W: Hearing by cochlear nucleus stimulation in humans. Ann Otol Rhinol Laryngol Suppl 1982;91:117–124.
2   Eisenberg LS, Maltan AA, Portillo F, Mobley JP, House WF: Electrical stimulation of the auditory brain stem structure in deafened adults. J Rehab Res Dev 1987;24:9–22.
3   Portillo F, Nelson RA, Brackmann DE, et al: Auditory brain stem implant: electrical stimulation of the human cochlear nucleus. Adv Otorhinolaryngol 1993;48:248–252.
4   Brackmann DE, Hitselberger WE, Nelson RA, et al: Auditory brainstem implant. I. Issues in surgical implantation. Otolaryngol Head Neck Surg 1993;108:624–633.
5   Shannon RV, Fayad J, Moore J, et al: Auditory brainstem implant. II. Postsurgical issues and performance. Otolaryngol Head Neck Surg 1993;108:634–642.
6   Schwartz MS, Otto SR, Brackmann DE, Hitselberger WE, Shannon RV: Use of a multichannel auditory brainstem implant for neurofibromatosis type 2. Stereotact Funct Neurosurg 2003;81:110–114.
7   Otto SR, Brackmann DE, Hitselberger WE, Shannon RV, Kuchta J: Multichannel auditory brainstem implant: update on performance in 61 patients. J Neurosurg 2002;96:1063–1071.
8   Otto SR, Brackmann DE, Hitselberger W: Auditory brainstem implantation in 12- to 18-year-olds. Arch Otolaryngol Head Neck Surg 2004;130:656–659.
9   Nevison B, Laszig R, Sollmann WP, et al: Results from a European clinical investigation of the Nucleus multichannel auditory brainstem implant. Ear Hear 2002;23:170–183.
10 Colletti V, Carner M, Miorelli V, Guida M, Colletti L, Fiorino F: Auditory brainstem implant (ABI): new frontiers in adults and children. Otolaryngol Head Neck Surg 2005;133:126–138.
11 Colletti V, Shannon RV: Open set speech perception with auditory brainstem implant? Laryngoscope 2005;115:1974–1978.
12 Colletti V, Sacchetto L, Giarbini N, Fiorino F, Carner M: Retrosigmoid approach for auditory brainstem implant. J Laryngol Otol Suppl 2000:37–40.
13 Terr LI, Edgerton BJ: Surface topography of the cochlear nuclei in humans: two and three-dimensional analysis. Hear Res 1985;17:51–59.
14 Kuroki A, Møller AR: Microsurgical anatomy around the foramen of Luschka with reference to intraoperative recording of auditory evoked potentials from the cochlear nuclei. J Neurosurg 1995;82:933–939.

15 Waring MD: Intraoperative electrophysiologic monitoring to assist placement of auditory brain stem implant. Ann Otol Rhinol Laryngol Suppl 1995;166:33–36.
16 Heller JW, Brackmann DE, Tucci DL, Nyenhuis JA, Chou CK: Evaluation of MRI compatibility of the modified nucleus multichannel auditory brainstem and cochlear implants. Am J Otol 1996;17:724–729.

Jose N. Fayad, MD
House Clinic
2100 West Third Street
Los Angeles, CA 90057 (USA)
Tel. +1 213 353 7093, Fax +1 213 484 5900, E-Mail jfayad@hei.org

Møller AR (ed): Cochlear and Brainstem Implants.
Adv Otorhinolaryngol. Basel, Karger, 2006, vol 64, pp 154–166

....

A Guide to the Positioning of Brainstem Implants Using Intraoperative Electrical Auditory Brainstem Responses

Barry Nevison

Cochlear Europe Ltd., Addlestone, UK

Abstract

The number of electrodes that elicit usable auditory sensations with an auditory brainstem implant varies significantly between subjects. For those with only very few, movement of the array by only a few millimetres could make a significant improvement to their outcome, but yet the point at which this is normally discovered is during activation, weeks after the surgery. The number of the electrodes that are able to stimulate the auditory system can be more reliably assured by the use of electrophysiologic guidance in the placement of the implanted electrode array. This chapter describes a procedure for the use of electrophysiology to aid placement in the operating room. The procedure involves stimulating the individual electrodes and recording electrical auditory brainstem responses (EABR) as an aid in positioning the electrode array. This procedure makes it possible to position the majority of electrodes over the surface of the cochlear nucleus thus minimising stimulation of other cranial nerves, which might result in undesirable side effects. Correctly positioned electrodes elicit an EABR response with between 1 and 4 peaks with average latencies approximately (in ms) 0.7 (0.4–0.9), 1.5 (1.2–1.9), 2.7 (2.1–3.4) and 3.7 (3.4–4.0). These waves likely correspond to waves III–VI of the traditional ABR (and wave II if an excitable stump of the auditory nerve is present). No further peaks within a 10-ms window should be seen nor should activation of other cranial nerves occur. The response to stimulation of bipolar combinations of electrodes covering lateral, medial and distal positions provide information about the insertion depth. In individuals with a large lateral recess, measuring other combinations may assist in sideways and rotational orientation of the electrode array.

Copyright © 2006 S. Karger AG, Basel

Over 90% of recipients of an auditory brainstem implant (ABI) experience some kind of side effects as revealed during psychophysical testing to create their hearing program [1]. Obviously the purpose of the fitting process is to give

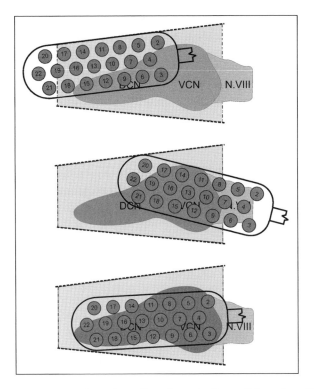

Fig. 1. Illustration of how theoretically small lateral, medial and rotational positions of the ABI array could affect coverage over the excitable CN complex in a large lateral recess.

the patient a hearing program which is only auditory and this is usually achieved, but different recipients have vastly different numbers of usable electrodes – from the unfortunate cases where this is zero, to those cases where every electrode may be used. When all, or nearly all electrodes give auditory sensations, it can be assumed that whatever result the patient achieves is the best possible result. When perhaps only a quarter of the electrode array gives auditory sensations it seems likely that a slightly different position might have given this recipient a better outcome, and moving the array by a few millimetres in one direction or the other could have made a great difference in outcome (fig. 1). When this is discovered post-surgery repositioning of the array is impossible. It is therefore important to use electrophysiological guidance during the operation where it is possible to adjust the position of the electrode array. The approximate size of the exposed cochlear nucleus (CN) surface closely matches the dimensions of the Nucleus 24 ABI electrode array (8.5×3.0 mm), but unlike a cochlear implant surgery, there are no solid structures upon which to demark the exact periphery of the CN complex, only bulges, veins, colourations, stumps, adjacent nerve groups and surrounding structures which lead to the opening of the lateral recess [2]. Since the full surface of the CN is not visible, even the experienced surgeon may have difficulties in placement of the electrode array into an optimal position every time. Distorted anatomy caused by the removal of a large tumour, or 'normal' anatomical variations makes the task even more difficult. Electrophysiologic guidance can reduce these problems [3]. The less experienced surgeon will have even greater help from electrophysiology.

In some situations the electrophysiological guidance (using recordings of the EARB during placement of the electrode array) may confirm optimal placement, while in other situations the results will show that the electrode array needs a slightly different orientation or depth into the lateral recess of the fourth ventricle.

This paper provides information about the use of recordings of evoked potentials as a guide for placement of the electrode array on the surface of the CN for optimal performance of ABIs.

Intraoperative Recording of the Electrical Auditory Brainstem Response

The acoustic auditory brainstem response (ABR) (fig. 2) of an individual with normal hearing is characterized by 5–7 vertex-positive waves that normally occur within the first 6–7 ms after a click or tone pip stimulus delivered to the ear. These peaks that are labelled by Roman numerals are generated by the auditory nerve (peak I and II) and fibres and nerve cells in the ascending auditory pathways (peak III onwards). It is generally assumed that peak III of the ABR is generated by the CN and peak V is generated by the lateral lemniscus where it terminates in the inferior colliculus, and that the slow negative deflection that follows peak V is generated by cells and dendrites of the inferior colliculus [4]. The electrically evoked ABR (EABR) [5] elicited by electrical stimulation of the CN (fig. 2) is similar to the ABR but does not contain components that correspond to peak I or peak II (usually). The latencies of the peaks (when adjusted for the different activation sites) that are generated in the CN and the lateral lemniscus are shorter than those of the ABR (fig. 2) and also slightly different to those of a cochlear implant EABR (fig. 2, table 1). The reason that there may be a component that corresponds to peak II of the ABR could be due to stimulation of the proximal stump of the auditory nerve that is functional a short time after implantation. When these fibres have degenerated one would not expect to see this component remain in the EABR.

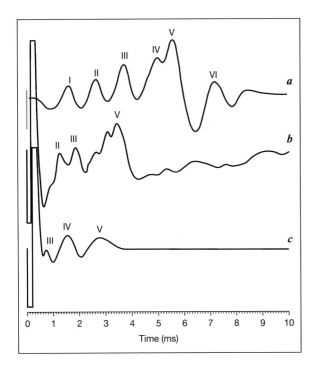

Fig. 2. The ABR illustration: acoustic ABR (***a***), electrical EABR from a CI recipient (***b***), electrical EABR from an ABI recipient (***c***).

Table 1. Typical acoustic ABR and EABR latencies in adults

Wave	Acoustic ABR typical peak latency, ms	Electrical EABR typical peak latency (CI), ms
I	1.6	(buried in stimulus)
II	2.7	1.3
III	3.7	2.0
IV	4.9	–
V	5.6	3.5
VI	6.9	5.5

Electrical stimulation of the CN complex may cause a different pattern of activation than that caused by the input from the auditory nerve affecting the latencies and amplitudes and peaks in the EABR. The fact that most patients who receive an ABI have neurofibromatosis type 2 may also affect the function of the CN and thus the electrical activity that is generated.

Use of EABR to Guide Positioning of the Electrode Array

Intraoperative electrophysiology during ABI surgery serves to demonstrate that electrical stimulation from the implanted electrode array elicits a response from the ascending auditory pathway as reflected in the recorded EABR. Monitoring of neighbouring cranial nerves serves to detect activity that indicates misplacement of the electrode array. This chapter will concentrate on monitoring of the EABR for guiding electrode placement.

Equipment Requirements

Although a single machine could suffice for recording EABR and cranial nerve monitoring, it may be advantageous to use separate equipment for monitoring the cranial nerves V, VII, IX and X and for recording the EABR waveforms. For monitoring cranial nerves, bipolar needle electrodes are placed in muscles that are innervated by each one.

An electrode montage described by Waring [6] is used for EABR during ABI surgery. This uses vertex (Cz) as positive, neck hairline (on the midline) as ground, C7 (on the spine, midline) as negative. Short, platted or twisted recording electrode wires are used to reduce electrical interference. The electrode wires are connected directly into an electrode head-box that is connected to the main amplifier.

The electrode montage for EABR during ABI operations is different from that used for recording regular ABR or cochlear implant EABR, which typically uses vertex (Cz) or upper forehead as positive, ipsilateral mastoid as ground, contralateral mastoid as negative. The use of the traditional ABR montage for recording an EABR, both with ABI and CI, will result in a larger stimulus artifact than the montage described above.

The electrical stimulus generates a large potential immediately preceding the neural response. This has two specific complicating effects: (1) The stimulus artifact may extend in time and overlap with the response. (2) The amplitude of the stimulus (which is orders of magnitude greater than the response) may cause the amplifiers to become overloaded or 'saturated', obscuring any response which should occur within the first milliseconds after the stimulus. Both of the above phenomena can be managed by a combination of: (a) electrode montage, (b) filtering, (c) gain settings, and (d) stimulus control.

It is preferable not to filter the input signal as much as when recording ABR. Filter cut-offs should be in the 1–10 Hz range (high-pass filter) to 5–10 kHz (low-pass filter) range. Too high a setting of the high-pass filter, for example to 100 Hz or above, can adversely affect the recording, as shown in figure 3 which shows the

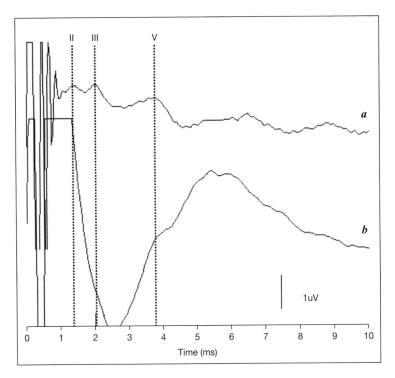

Fig. 3. Affect of HP filter on stimulus artifact, shown here for an EABR recorded with a cochlear implant recipient. HP = 10 Hz (***a***) and 100 Hz (***b***).

same cochlear implant EABR recording with 10- and 100-Hz cut-offs. The way filtering affects the stimulus artifact depends on the type of filters used. The use of zero-phase finite impulse response digital filters can prevent the smearing of the stimulus artifact in time [7].

Saturation of the amplifiers can be controlled by using modest gain settings, which are a compromise between that needed to sufficiently amplify the response above the noise whilst not excessively amplifying the stimulus artifact. A $\pm 100\,mV$ stimulus artifact amplified by $\times 1,000$ (equals 100 V) will saturate an amplifier if its maximum output is 5 V. The same signal amplified by $\times 100$ will cause a much lesser degree of saturation. Different kinds of evoked potential equipment refer to the gain value differently. Some refer to the front-end amplifier gain only and then have a separate scaling for the display; others have a single value that directly influences the display scaling. When using modern systems, one might not need to worry so much about these problems because amplifier design has improved significantly in recent years and they are generally far more capable of recovering quickly from massive saturation.

Finally, the stimulus artifact depends on the intensity of the stimulus and the pulse width. The use of too wide pulses may obscure the response. The author has good experience using pulse widths in the range of 100–200 µs, rather than the default pulse widths, which are narrower.

The stimuli are generated by the ABI programming system, which also provides a trigger signal for the evoked potential machine that is used for EABR recordings. Typically, approximately 1,000 responses must be averaged to achieve an acceptable signal to noise ratio. Post-stimulus delays should be set to 0 ms as it can be helpful to see the stimulus on the screen in order to better interpret the response. Other features such as artifact rejection can be enabled provided they are set not to reject anything within the first 2 ms after the stimulus.

Stimulation

The manufacturer's programming software will allow for set-up of the stimulus to be used during surgery. With the Nucleus 24 ABI system, this is achieved using their NRT 3.1 software, which has an EABR functionality feature. For EABR, rates of approximately 35 Hz are suitable. The sequence of tested electrodes shown in figure 4 provides information about insertion depth (mainly) and rotation. It is important to use bipolar electrode combinations. Monopolar stimulation creates much larger stimulus artifacts and may stimulate tissue other than the CN. The stimulus must be increased from a low starting intensity and increased until a clear multi-peaked EABR waveform is observed. The author's experience with the Nucleus ABI suggests starting with a pulse width of approximately 150 µs, and a current level of approximately 150 CL units in bipolar mode. Electrically this corresponds to a charge of approximately 30 nC. Normally this will be slightly below threshold, and a reliable response is usually obtained before reaching 220 CLs or 130 nC. Despite the small surface areas of the electrodes, these levels are still well within published safety data [8, 9]. The threshold provides a measure of the excitability of the CN complex. Lower thresholds indicate that the tested electrode is in a good position on the surface of the CN and that any adjacent structures are less likely to be stimulated.

Confirming the approximate placement of an electrode array is best achieved with a relatively wide bipolar stimulation path across most of the array (fig. 4a, b). The wider modes are more likely to stimulate nearby cranial nerves, which then can be detected provided that the cranial nerves in question are monitored. If this occurs with low stimulus current levels, it is a strong indication to change the position of the electrode array.

For more accurate placement of the electrode array, a combination of electrodes across the array should be stimulated (fig. 4c, d). Each position should

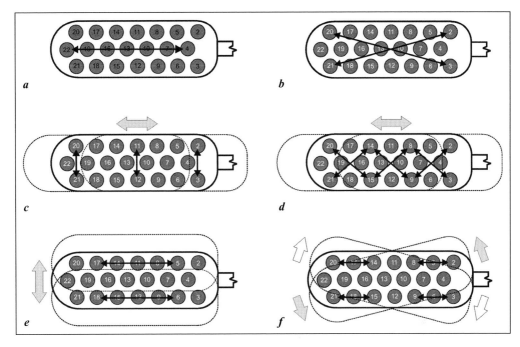

Fig. 4. Electrode stimulation options to assist in device positioning. *a, b* Gross positioning. *c, d* Lateral/medial shift. *e, f* Rotational/sideways shift.

be tested and the responses compared before making any decision about advancing or retracting the electrode array. Rotational and/or sideways positioning is far more difficult in practice because of the limited space available. In cases where the lateral recess is wide, combinations of electrodes along the sides of the array (fig. 4e, f) should be stimulated, since 1 mm of sub-optimal placement in this direction could make 7 electrodes non-functional compared to only 3 electrodes for incorrect placement in the lateral-medial direction.

After examining a response, the stimulus polarity should be inverted and a second response obtained, making sure that only the stimulus artifact inverts and not the response. When responses are small and noisy, this is the best indicator that the observed potential is biological and neither noise, stimulus artifacts nor an artifact of the filtering.

Stimulation at high current levels has the possibility to stimulate the vagus nerve and may cause heart arrest, which has occurred using current levels of approximately 150 nC in two cases. Cessation of stimulation caused sinus rhythm to return immediately. The anaesthesiologist should always be alerted to this possibility in order to keep additional attention to the vital signs.

Characterising the Response

The waveform of the recorded EABRs differ considerably among patients. From the author's experience of over 100 intraoperative recordings, normally between 1 and 4 positive waves can be identified within a window of approximately 4 ms from the start of the stimulus. No dominant component normally occurs in the remainder of the observation window (typically 10 ms). It is more common to see 2- or 3-peak responses than 1 or 4 peaks. The most dominant and reliable positive peak occurs at a latency of approximately 1.5 ms (1.2–1.9 ms). An earlier and often indistinct peak is occasionally visible at a latency of 0.4–0.9 ms. Later peaks occur often in the range of latencies between 2.2–4.0 ms. The early peak may be obscured or altered by the stimulus artifact or it may be an artifact of amplifier recovery. However, since a positive peak appears in response to both stimulus polarities, this early peak is believed to be of biological origin.

The average latencies of the peaks of the EABR fall within broad ranges (table 2), with or without all peaks necessarily being distinct. This individual variation might indicate that either different auditory pathways are activated in different patients or that the state of the auditory pathway differs among patients, and especially those who have a tumour or have had surgery to remove them. Nevertheless, these matters are not essential for the use of EABR recordings for positioning of the electrode array, provided it is possible to observe several peaks occurring within this 4-ms window. Any biological activity observed in the 5–10 ms window or any strong activity from the cranial nerves would suggest simultaneous activation of other structures than the CN.

Occurrence of distinct components within the 4-ms window is not always a sign of proper activation of the CN if, for example, there appears a sequence of peaks that look like sinusoidal waves with progressively smaller amplitudes. This could indicate an amplifier-related oscillation (as shown previously in fig. 3). Inverting the stimulus should cause the oscillation to invert if it is non-biological in origin.

If only a single peak occurs in the 4-ms window it may indicate activation of some neural tissue but no corresponding activation of ascending auditory pathways. A single peak could also mean correct positioning but poor synchrony of neurons in the CN, which would suggest lower expectations for the performance of the ABI. Figure 5a–c shows examples of intraoperative EABRs with 1–4 peaks, obtained from different ABI recipients.

There are many different sources of electrical interference in an operating room and electrical interference can obscure the recorded responses. For example, cautery/diathermy machines tend to produce interference even in standby. It is important that such interference is brought to a minimum before a recording is begun [for details about reducing electrical and magnetic interference, see 7].

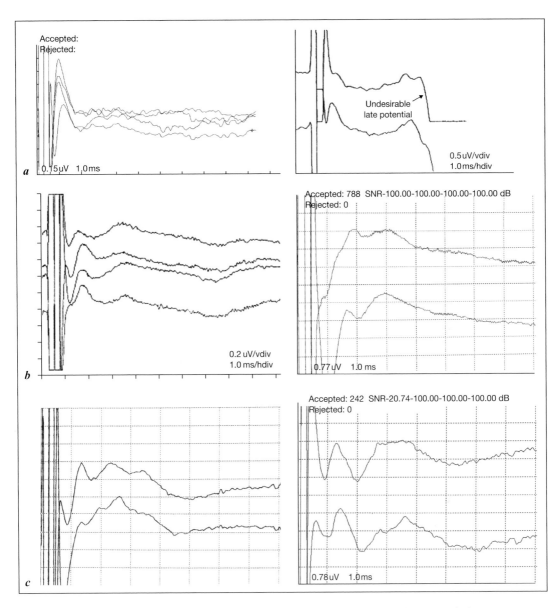

Fig. 5. Range of EABR responses recorded from ABI recipients intraoperatively: 1 peak (*a*), 2 or 3 peaks (*b*), 3 or 4 peaks (*c*).

Table 2. Average EABR latencies with an ABI

	Average EABR latency, ms	Range, ms
Peak 1	0.6	0.4–0.9
Peak 2	1.5	1.2–1.9
Peak 3	2.7	2.1–3.4
Peak 4	3.7	3.4–4.0

If the waveforms are saturated by a large, decaying stimulus artifact, consider widening the stimulus pulse width to lower the stimulus current requirements, lower the high-pass filter cut-off and reduce the amplification. Alternatively, try electrode combinations that have a different orientation to that initially chosen. If no clear response is observed by 150 nC, then it is unlikely that any technical action will bring a response to appear. Lack of excitability of the CN, inaccurate positioning of the electrode array or poor contact with the CN surface are likely causes of the failure to obtain a response. Repositioning or repacking behind the ABI array may be options to consider.

Discussion

The advantages of intraoperative electrophysiologic guidance in placement of ABI electrode arrays should not be underestimated. It might be argued that knowing the anatomy ensures correct placement of the electrode array and that multiple repositionings only risk traumatizing the CN complex, reducing eventual benefit. Even for the very experienced surgeon the reassurance that the EABR provides can be significant, especially if the anatomy has been distorted by a large tumour. Improving the position of the electrode array beyond that which can be assessed on purely anatomical grounds is likely to improve the performance of the ABI. For the less experienced surgeon, guidance through the use of recordings of EABR may make the difference between success and partial failure, necessitating re-operations. Proper placement of the electrode array also reduces the risk of non-auditory sensations when the ABI is in use.

Some investigators have described the use of ABI in patients with pathologies other than bilateral vestibular schwannoma, including young children with cochlear nerve aplasia [10–12]. This presents a different challenge regarding placement of the electrode array because of differences in the anatomy (e.g. the absence of an VIIIth nerve altogether). It also presents challenges in their device activation due to the reduced feedback about sound and side effect sensations. Here the role of EABR is possibly even more significant.

The use of Neural Response Telemetry for recording the neural activity from a location near the implanted electrode array may also be of value in electrode placement and during programming of ABI devices [13]. However, since the Neural Response Telemetry measures the near-field response and not any activity in the ascending pathway its use may be limited, as is the author's experience.

Conclusions

Intraoperative recording of EABR during implantation of the ABI electrode array provides the surgical team with information about the ability of the implanted electrodes to activate neurons in the CN. This information may be used to correct the position of the electrode array peri-operatively and offer reassurance at the end of the operation that the CN complex can be stimulated by as many electrodes as possible for the individual recipient.

Despite good intraoperative EABR, occasionally only few auditory electrodes may function post-operatively. This can be caused by movement of the electrode array after the operation or, in some cases, the stump of the VIIIth nerve may have given temporarily good EABRs in the operating room but after its atrophy the electrodes fail to stimulate. Monitoring of other cranial nerves may be helpful in implantation of an ABI electrode array. Such monitoring is always justified in operations for removal of vestibular schwannoma such as often precedes implantation of ABIs.

Acknowledgements

Grateful thanks to Martin O'Driscoll from Manchester Royal Infirmary, UK, for most of the 2-, 3- and 4-peak EABR sample waveforms.

References

1   Nevison B, Laszig R, Sollmann WP, Lenaz T, Sterkers O, Ramsden R, Fraysse B, Manrique M, Rask-Andersen H, Garcia-Ibanez E, Colletti V, von Wallenberg E: Results from a European clinical investigation of the Nucleus multichannel auditory brainstem implant. Ear Hear 2002;23:170–183.
2   Kuroki A, Møller AR: Microsurgical anatomy around the foramen of Luschka with reference to intraoperative recording of auditory evoked potentials from the cochlear nuclei. J Neurosurg 1995;933–939.
3   Waring MD: Intraoperative electrophysiologic monitoring to assist placement of auditory brain stem implant. Ann Otol Rhinol Laryngol Suppl 1995;166:33–36.

4   Møller AR: Hearing: Anatomy, Physiology and Disorders of the Auditory System, ed 2. Amsterdam, Elsevier, 2006.
5   Waring MD: Auditory brain-stem responses evoked by electrical stimulation of the cochlear nucleus in human subjects. Electroenceph Clin Neurophysiol 1995;96:338–347.
6   Waring MD: Properties of auditory brainstem responses evoked by intra-operative electrical stimulation of the cochlear nucleus in human subjects. Electroencephalogr Clin Neurophysiol 1996;100:538–548.
7   Møller AR: Intraoperative Neurophysiologic Monitoring, ed 2. Totowa, Humana Press, 2006.
8   McCreery DB, Agnew WF, Yuen TG, Bullara L: Charge density and charge per phase as cofactors in neural injury induced by electrical stimulation. IEEE Trans Biomed Eng 1990;37:996–1001.
9   Shannon RV: A model of safe levels for electrical stimulation. IEEE Trans Biomed Eng 1992;39: 424–426.
10   Colletti V, Carner M, Miorelli V, Guida M, Colletti L, Fiorino F: Auditory brainstem implant (ABI): new frontiers in adults and children. Otolaryngol Head Neck Surg 2005;133:126–138.
11   Colletti V, Carner M, Fiorino F, Sacchetto L, Miorelli V, Orsi A, Cilurzo F, Pacini L: Hearing restoration with auditory brainstem implant in three children with cochlear nerve aplasia. Otol Neurotol 2002;23:682–693.
12   Colletti V, Fiorino F, Sacchetto L, Miorelli V, Carner M: Hearing habilitation with auditory brainstem implantation in two children with cochlear nerve aplasia. Int J Pediatr Otorhinolaryngol 2001;60:99–111.
13   Otto S, Waring M, Kuchta J: Neural response telemetry and auditory/nonauditory sensations in 15 recipients of auditory brainstem implants. J Am Acad Audiol 2005;16:219–227.

Barry Nevison, BEng DPhil
Cochlear Europe Ltd., 9 Weybridge Business Park
Addlestone Road
Addlestone KT15 2UF (UK)
Tel. +44 1932 871500, Fax +44 1932 871526, E-Mail bnevison@cochlear.co.uk

Møller AR (ed): Cochlear and Brainstem Implants.
Adv Otorhinolaryngol. Basel, Karger, 2006, vol 64, pp 167–185

....

Auditory Outcomes in Tumor vs. Nontumor Patients Fitted with Auditory Brainstem Implants

Vittorio Colletti

Clinica ORL, Ospedale Policlinico, Verona, Italy

Abstract

Auditory brainstem implants (ABIs) are currently indicated for patients older than 12 years with neurofibromatosis type 2 (NF2) who had bilateral schwannoma removed. Over the last 10 years, we have extended the indications for ABIs to nontumor children and adult patients with cochlear or cochlear nerve injuries or malfunctions who would not benefit from a cochlear implant. We have provided ABIs for patients with cochlear nerve aplasia and other injuries, and patients in whom any benefit was, or would be, severely compromised as in extensive cochlear ossification. In the present chapter we report our recent findings in adult ABI patients and compare the psychophysical and speech perception outcomes in tumor with those in nontumor patients. We demonstrate that the ABI can stimulate the central auditory system in a way that gives the ability of open set speech understanding, and can thus be indicated in nontumor adult patients who are not candidates for a cochlear implant. From April 1997 to January 2006, a total of 80 patients, 62 adults and 18 children, were fitted with ABIs in the University of Verona ENT Department; age ranged from 14 months to 70 years. Twenty-six patients had NF2 with bilateral vestibular schwannoma removal, and 54 had nontumor diseases of the cochlear nerve or cochlea. The retrosigmoid approach was used in all patients. All patients had a functioning implantation, and no complications were observed during the operation, activation as well as long-term use of the ABI. All patients, except 1 (NF2), reported auditory sensations with activation of various numbers of electrodes (from 5 to 21). Different electrodes elicited different pitch sensations. At 1 year after implantations nontumor adults scored from 12 to 100% in open set speech perception tests (average 59%), and tumor (NF2) patients scored from 5 to 30% (average of 11%). The differences between these results are statistically significantly ($p < 0.01$). To investigate the cause of the differences in performance between tumor and nontumor ABI recipients, a series of psychophysical tests were done consecutively in 39 adult patients with implants (25 nontumor and 14 tumor patients) from May 1999 to April 2004 and with a follow-up of at least 1 year. The outcome of this study shows that: (1) The ABIs allow most tumor and nontumor patients to experience improved communication as well as awareness of environmental sounds. (2) Nontumor patients had better hearing outcomes than tumor patients when the variation in the auditory benefit with the ABI in relation to the patient's underlying pathological conditions were taken into consideration. (3) A significant number of nontumor patients are able understand speech at a level comparable to that of the most successful cochlear implant users including conversational telephone use. (4) The ABI represents the tool for hearing rehabilitation in patients with profound hearing loss who cannot be fitted with cochlear implants.

Approximately 400 neurofibromatosis type 2 (NF2) patients have received multichannel auditory brainstem implants (ABIs) worldwide, and obtained a functionally beneficial level of auditory input to assist them with their communication needs. Patients with other diseases involving the cochlear nerve or the cochlea, with a similar disconnection of the central auditory systems from sound, have so far not been considered to be candidates for treatment with an ABI. The cochlear nerve may be congenitally absent, or destroyed due to acquired disorders (e.g. posttraumatic cochlear nerve avulsion) or, the cochlea may be so severely compromised that fitting of a cochlear implant becomes difficult, inappropriate, or even impossible as is the case with cochlear aplasia, and postmeningitis cochlear ossification. In view of the site and the nature of such lesions and the ability of modern ABI devices to provide stimulation directly to the first central auditory station (cochlear nucleus-CN), it is surprising that the indications for the ABI have been limited to tumor patients. Indeed, lack of intervention condemns such individuals to a dramatic inability to communicate. Fear of unsatisfactory auditory results, risk of complications, surgical limitations and ethical reasons were, and probably still are, the reasons for limiting the indication of ABIs to patients with NF2 [1–3]. For a detailed analysis and discussion of these issues, see Colletti et al. [4].

One major reason why the use of ABIs was restricted to patients with NF2 and who had had bilateral vestibular schwannoma removed is probably that the ABI yields poor hearing results, and certainly not comparable to those which can be achieved with cochlear implants. The overall ABI performance in such tumor patients is in fact no better than that achieved by single-channel cochlear implants, whereas multichannel cochlear implants can restore speech understanding to a level where most patients can converse on the telephone. However, in view of the worldwide acceptance of the use of ABI in such patients, it must be assumed that the improvement in communication skills through the use of ABIs in patients with NF2 is not negligible. This is supported by the progressive increase in the number of centers providing ABIs. In Europe, the number of centers that treat NF2 patients with ABIs has increased from 9 in 1998 to 22 in 2005. Absence of a significant improvement in communication skills from ABIs in such patients must have rapidly discouraged its application with a decline of interest in the device.

In this paper we review our recent findings in the use of ABI, and we compare the outcome of psychophysical and speech perception tests in tumor patients with that obtained in nontumor patients. We present evidence that ABIs can provide sufficient stimulation of the central auditory system for open set speech understanding to justify the extension of the indication to patients without tumors.

Methods

Patients

From April 1997 to January 2006 a total of 80 patients (62 adults and 18 children; age range: 14 months to 70 years) were fitted with ABIs in the ENT Department of the University of Verona. These patients were suffering from tumors of the cerebellopontine angle (26 patients) and from a variety of nontumor diseases (54 patients) of the cochlea or cochlear nerve. The retrosigmoid-transmeatal approach was used in tumor patients and the retrosigmoid approach in all nontumor patients. Seventy patients (16 tumor and 54 nontumor) were fitted with a Nucleus 24 Cochlear ABI (Cochlear Co., Lane Cove, Australia), 6 tumor patients were fitted with a Nucleus 21 Cochlear ABI (Cochlear Co.); 1 nontumor and 3 tumor patients received a Med-El Pulsar ci100 ABI (Med-El Co., Innsbruck, Austria).

Twenty-six patients, 20 adults and 2 children, had NF2 with bilateral vestibular schwannoma removed, and 4 adults had solitary unilateral vestibular schwannoma in the only hearing ear. Ten children had bilateral cochlear nerve aplasia; four with associated cochlear malformations, two with associated unilateral facial nerve agenesis and 1 with combined microtia and aural atresia. Two of these children had been fitted with a cochlear implant elsewhere. Two adults and 3 children presented with cochlear malformations. One child, who had previously been fitted unsuccessfully with a cochlear implant, and 2 adults had auditory neuropathy. One child and 29 adults showed bilaterally altered cochlear patency: 17 patients had complete bilateral cochlear ossification, and 13 patients presented with cochlear derangement of the turns caused by meningitis (7), otosclerosis (15), or autoimmune disease (8). Four adults of this group had not received any benefit from a previously fitted cochlear implant. Six patients, 5 adults and 1 child, had profound hearing loss after head trauma with different degrees of cochlear fractures. For a detailed description of the patient population, see Colletti et al. [4–8].

To investigate differences in performances between tumor and nontumor patients, 39 adult ABI patients (25 nontumor and 14 patients with NF2 who had had bilateral vestibular schwannoma removed), were selected for a series of psychophysical tests. These patients were operated upon consecutively from May 1999 to April 2004. The sizes of the tumors ranged from 4 to 52 mm: 4 tumors were judged to be small, 5 medium and 5 large (fig. 1). The 25 nontumor patients had different types of diseases; 4 patients had bilateral labyrinthine fractures (fig. 2a), 1 had a bilateral temporal bone fracture, 2 had cochlear malformations characterized by incomplete cochlear partition (type II or Mondini malformations; fig. 2b), 18 had different alteration of the cochlear patency, 10 had complete bilateral cochlear ossification (fig. 2c) and 8 presented with cochlear derangement of the turns (fig. 2d) due to meningitis (3 patients), otosclerosis (2) and autoimmune diseases (3). Two of these patients had been previously fitted with a cochlear implant elsewhere.

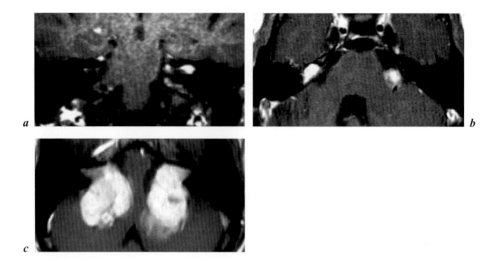

Fig. 1. Encephalic MRIs with gadolinium enhancement showing CPA tumors of different sizes. *a* Small tumors in coronal view. *b* Medium tumors in axial plane. *c* Large tumors in axial plane; the large bilateral tumors compress the brainstem.

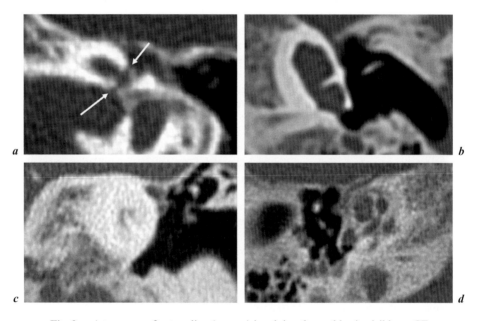

Fig. 2. *a* A transverse fracture line (arrows) involving the cochlea is visible on CT scan in axial view. *b* CT scan shows in coronal view an incomplete cochlear partition (type II or Mondini malformation). *c* A left complete cochlear ossification (T.L.; for details, see text) is evident on CT scan (coronal view). *d* CT scan (coronal view) shows a cochlear derangement.

Approval of the study was obtained from the ethical Committee of the University of Verona Hospital, and the patients gave informed consent for the implantation and the subsequent studies.

The auditory performances of the patients that were selected for this study were comparable with those obtained in the remaining ABI population for both tumor and nontumor patients. Average open-set sentence recognition score in the auditory only mode obtained 1 year after implantation was 6% in the tested tumor group, 11% in the remaining tumor patients (p = n.s.), 46% in the tested nontumor group, and 59% in the remaining nontumor patients (p = n.s.).

Description of the ABI Devices

A Nucleus 21 Cochlear ABI was used in the first 6 patients who received implants. It was based on the Nucleus 22-channel Cochlear Implant System. It had a silicone elastomer electrode carrier 8.5 mm long, 3.0 mm wide and 0.6 mm thick. Twenty-one platinum disk electrodes, 0.7 mm in diameter, arranged in three diagonally offset rows were on one face of this carrier. The electrodes were connected to a Nucleus cochlear implant 22 M* receiver-stimulator by a silicone elastomer lead 1.2 mm in diameter and 11 cm long containing 21 individually insulated, helically wound, 25-μm platinum/iridium (90/10%) wires. A special narrow-weave mesh cut into the shape of the letter T was attached to the rear surface of the carrier with the aim to promote fibrous tissue growth helping and fixing the array in situ. It had one reference electrode. The receiver/stimulator was identical to the Nucleus 22 M cochlear implant with a single monopolar plate electrode added to the top surface electronics capsule. A Spectra 22 speech processor controlled the stimulation [9]. The Nucleus 24 cochlear ABI is based on the nucleus 24 M cochlear implant systems.

The Nucleus 24 cochlear ABI has been used since 1999 and differs from the Nucleus 22 ABI in its possibility to use different stimulation strategies, and to utilize the neural response telemetry for performing intraoperative electrical monitoring of the neural interface, and the possibility of removing the magnet from the internal receiver/stimulator of the device.

The use of the neural response telemetry that provides a near-field monitoring of evoked potentials from the cochlear nucleus might be useful in verifying the correct positioning of the ABI in the lateral recess and to define the stimulus level to be used at ABI activation. This should be particularly advantageous in children.

The Nucleus 24 cochlear ABI has speech processing strategies such as continuous interleaved sampling and advanced combination encoder (ACE), see Introduction and the paper by Loizou [this vol, pp 109–143]. The impulses that are delivered to the implanted electrodes with the SPEAK strategy have a modest rate of 250–300 pulses/s (pps). The number and location of the electrodes to be stimulated are selected based on the intensity and frequency of the incoming signal. The continuous interleaved sampling strategy employs a high fixed rate of stimulation (600–1,800 pps) delivered to a small number of channels. The ACE strategy combines the advantages of both the SPEAK and cochlear implant strategies. It has a high rate of stimulation (600–1,800 pps), a large dynamic electrode selection and numerous available electrodes, improving the transmission of temporal and spectral speech information. For further discussion of processor strategies, see Introduction and the paper by Loizou [this vol, pp 109–143].

The electrode array of the Nucleus 24 cochlear ABI device has a flat silicone carrier (3 × 8 mm), where the 21 platinum electrodes are arranged in 3 rows and 3 electrodes as reference. The individual electrode diameter is 0.7 mm. A T-shaped Dacron mesh is attached to the electrode carrier to stabilize the device intraoperatively and to permit tissue growth for further postoperative stabilization.

Implantable portions of the Med-El Pulsar ci100 ABI consist of a processor with a stimulus generator, the active electrode array, and the reference electrode. The stimulator measures approximately 3.5×2.4 cm and is less than 0.4 mm thick. All electronic components are contained in a compact ceramic case. It consists of the implant circuitry and a powerful microchip that is encapsulated in the hermetically sealed ceramic housing. The implant housing and electronics of the ABI are identical to those of the C40+ cochlear implant (Med-El Co.). The ABI can process large amounts of data and it can provide updated information in each pulse at a high rate of up to 18,180 pps. This capability makes the stimulator compatible with a wide range of pulsatile coding strategies for future developments in speech processing. Telemetry features enable device function to be analyzed within seconds. Telemetry can assist in confirming the correct functioning of the implant and provide additional information that may be useful for programming the external speech processor. Information provided by telemetry includes impedances of the individual electrodes, ground path impedance, electrode status, voltage distribution, identification of short-circuits, and overall implant integrity.

The implanted electrode array of the Med-El Pulsar ci100 ABI consists of 12 active platinum contacts that are partially embedded in a flat oval-shaped silicone paddle. Soft and preshaped, the paddle is designed to fit onto the curved surface of the floor of the lateral recess of the brainstem. A polyester mesh embedded in silicone exceeds the size of the paddle, allowing tissue growth that will stabilize the electrode array onto the surface of the brainstem, thus minimizing the possibility of electrode movement or migration. The diameter of the electrode lead increases from 0.7 mm at the silicone paddle to 1.3 mm over a length of 10 mm.

Postoperative Procedures

Patients were followed postoperatively in the intensive care unit and returned to the ENT Department the day after the operation. CT scans were performed to evaluate electrode placement before discharge. Imaging showed the ABI in the proper position and no displacement occurred in any of the patients. On average, patients were hospitalized for 6 days after implantation. The ABIs were activated approximately 4–6 weeks after implantation. Because of the possible risks involved in stimulating brainstem structures, activation was done in the intensive care unit with electrocardiographic monitoring and with an anesthesiologist present.

Complications and Unwanted Effects of Stimulation

No complications were observed during the operation or on activation or during long-term use of the ABI in any of the patients who received implants. One patient (H.K.) who had extensive brainstem compression from multiple tumors (fig. 3), reported no auditory sensations, while other patients had

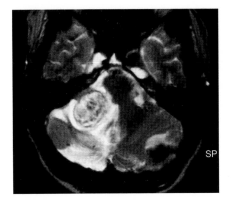

Fig. 3. Gadolinium-enhanced encephalic MRI demonstrating in the axial plane multiple tumors in the only patient (H.K.) with no auditory sensation at ABI activation. Extensive compression and displacement of the brainstem are evident.

auditory sensations for activation of 5–21 electrodes. The number of electrodes the activation of which induced nonauditory sensations varied from 1 to 8 among the patients. These electrodes were inactivated. Side effects were noted in 57 of 62 patients. The most common side effect was transitory dizziness that occurred in 47 patients. Tingling sensations in the leg, arm and throat were reported by 9, 7 and 4 patients, respectively (fig. 4). No contralateral side effects were observed. These nonauditory sensations often decreased in magnitude over time, and in 9 patients the electrodes that initially were associated with such side effects could be reactivated at a later session.

Results at the Time of Activation of the ABI

At activation, all patients except one (H.K.) could detect and recognize environmental sounds. Activation of different electrodes elicited different pitch sensations. A substantial variability of perceptual performance was characteristic for the group of patients we studied. This was true of all the different tests performed (closed-set vowel and consonant confusion test, closed-set word recognition, open-set sentence recognition and speech-tracking responses in the auditory mode alone and in the visual-auditory mode). These observations in ABI users are thus similar to the experience of cochlear implants where the results also vary greatly between individuals without the reason being known (see Introduction).

Processor Fitting and Programming

The protocol used for the activation and testing of the ABI and the evaluation of the auditory results differed between adults and children and has been detailed

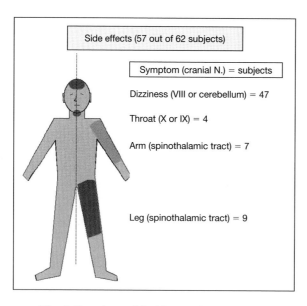

Fig. 4. Location and incidence of nonauditory side effects after ABI activation. For description, see text.

elsewhere [4–5]. Briefly, the threshold level and maximum comfortable levels of each electrode were first assessed to select the optimal electrode configuration. The monopolar mode was initially utilized to identify the electrodes that elicit auditory sensations. Electrodes that induce unpleasant sounds or nonauditory effects were excluded from future use. To determine an ABI recipient's perception of pitch and to define the appropriate tonotopic order of the electrodes, the place-pitch scaling and ranking procedures [4–5] were used. The processor was then programmed according to the pitch scaling and ranking results were obtained. On average, for the first 6 months from activation, the SPEAK encoder strategy was applied in all patients using the Investigational Protocol for the Clinical Trial of the Multichannel Auditory Brainstem Implant [10]. When the patients reach an auditory performance level without any improvement for 3 months, i.e. a 'plateau phase', the ACE strategy is utilized. ACE processors have higher stimulation rates, which allows better spectral and temporal resolution of speech signals and improvement in open-set speech recognition scores within a short period of time [11].

Follow-Up Tests

Patients were followed regularly for assessment of the efficacy and safety of their implants. Patients returned to our center for medical follow-up at 1 month,

6 months, and 1 year after activation and annually thereafter for reprogramming of their speech processors, and speech perception testing.

The following tests were performed:

(1) Recognition of environmental sound or sound detection test;
(2) Closed-set vowel confusion test;
(3) Closed-set consonant confusion test;
(4) Closed-set word recognition in the vision-only mode (lip-reading), sound-only mode, and sound-plus-vision mode;
(5) Open-set sentence recognition in the vision-only mode, sound-only mode, and sound-plus-vision mode;
(6) Speech-tracking test.

Speech Perception Evaluation

Postoperative auditory performance assessment is based on a battery of appropriate closed- and open-set measures included in the *Common Protocol of Evaluation of Audiological Rehabilitation Results*, which is an Italian version of *The Manual of Auditory Rehabilitation* [12]. Patients are seated 1 m in front of a speaker in a monitored common sound-field environment (a phonometer is used). Monitored live voice presentation with an intensity level of 70 dB HL is chosen for these tests in all patients because of the direct contact with the patient, allowing maintenance of the level of attention and vigilance. The tests are performed by the same person using the same speech material in each test session.

The closed-set vowel confusion test consists of 10 monosyllable vowels, composed of 5 long (BAAT, GAAT) and 5 short (BAT, GAT) words, delivered by live voice 4 times. The closed-set consonant confusion test is based on the delivery of 13 meaningless consonant words (ABA, AGA, ATA) read for the patients 4 times by live voice.

In the closed-set word recognition test, the speaker covers his face with a piece of paper and pronounces a word from among 12 words written on a list presented to the patient. The patient has to understand the word and repeat a word selected from the list of possible alternatives. In the open-set sentence recognition test, sentences on common topics are presented without providing a list of alternatives or other information to help identify the material. The results are scored in terms of the number of words or sentences that are correctly repeated by the patients.

In the speech-tracking test, a story is read to the patient (live voice), and the patient is supposed to repeat the sentences or words correctly. The number of correct words per minute in a 5-min session is determined. The sentences present different levels of difficulty. The score for normal-hearing individuals in this test is between 70 and 80 words per minute.

Results of Tests Performed 1 Year Postoperatively

Speech Tests

The results of closed-set word recognition, open-set sentence recognition in the auditory mode alone at 1 year for the total adult population are described below. When tested using the closed-set auditory alone mode, word recognition at 1 year after implantation for nontumor adults ranged from 40 to 100% (average 84%; median 80%). In the group of adults who had tumors removed, word recognition obtained in the same way and at the same time after implantation ranged from 5 to 41%, (average 25%; median 24%). The results from the tumor group are significantly lower ($p < 0.01$) than those observed in nontumor patients. On auditory alone mode, sentence recognition at 1 year ranged from 12 to 100% (average 59%; median 53%) in the nontumor group and from 5 to 30% (average 11%; median 16%) in the adult tumor group. These values were significantly lower ($p < 0.01$) in the nontumor subgroup compared with the tumor group.

Average and standard deviation of recognition scores for vowels were 37.4% (32.0) and 16.9% (15.5) for nontumor and NF2 patients, respectively. The difference was statistically significant ($p < 0.01$). Average and standard deviation of recognition scores for sentences were 27.4% (36.1) and 3.6% (6.2) for nontumor and NF2 patients, respectively, and the difference was statistically significant ($p < 0.005$; table 1). The correlation between average modulation detection threshold and sentence recognition ($r = -0.54$) was significant as was the correlation between modulation detection and vowel recognition ($r = -0.56$).

Word recognition in patients with head trauma, determined in closed-set auditory alone mode, ranged from 49 to 85%, patients with auditory neuropathy scored 40 and 46%, respectively, the two patients with cochlear malformations scored 58 and 60%, respectively, and patients with altered cochlear patency scored from 43 to 100%. At open set speech perception test, the patients with head trauma scored from 32 to 80%, the patients with auditory neuropathy scored 12 and 18%, respectively, the patients with cochlear malformations scored 57 and 61%, respectively, and patients with altered cochlear patency scored between 34 and 100%.

Electrical Threshold

Average threshold to electrical stimulation and standard deviation values for nontumor and NF2 patients were not significantly different: 12.6 (29.7) and 8.6 (12.4), respectively, and nontumor ABI patients (who had excellent speech recognition) and NF2 ABI patients (with poor speech recognition) had similar thresholds. These findings indicated good electrode placement and good survival of excitable neurons in both groups. Thresholds as low as 1.3 nC were

Table 1. Average, standard deviation and statistical outcomes of the psychophysical and speech results obtained for NF2 and nontumor patients

	Sentence recognition score, %	Vowel recognition score, %	Average modulation dB	Electrical threshold nC	Selectivity mm
Nontumor patients (n = 25)					
Average	27.47	37.43	−22.7	12.56	1.99
SD	36.06	31.98	9.0	29.73	0.99
Tumor patients (n = 14)					
Average	3.64	16.89	−13.98	8.63	1.17
SD	6.24	15.49	6.09	12.42	0.59
t test[1]	0.0017	0.0006	0.0053	0.2839	0.0518

[1]Nontumor vs. tumor patients.

observed, indicating that the distance between electrodes and cochlear nucleus neurons could be less than 1 mm [13, 14].

Electrode Selectivity

The distance at which the interference decreased by 1 dB from the maximum masking was used to quantify electrode selectivity. The average selectivity and its standard deviation were 2.0 (1.0) and 1.2 (0.6) for non-tumor and NF2 patients, respectively. Electrode selectivity measured in that way did not significantly correlate with vowel recognition or sentence recognition. Patients with excellent speech comprehension could have relatively poor selectivity, and patients with poor speech understanding could have excellent electrode selectivity.

Discrimination of Environmental Sounds

Environmental sounds were administered at ABI activation, and speech perception tests were performed 1 month, 6 months, and 1 year after activation; the speech-tracking test was administered in the patients who had a word recognition score of at least 50%. In the NF2 patients who were operated on on the first side, the contralateral ear with residual hearing was masked by delivering noise through a headphone. The masking noise consisted of broadband (Gaussian) noise presented continuously 10 dB above the patient's hearing threshold. When the patients visited the hospital, special attention was paid to the occurrence and magnitude of any nonauditory effects, such as dizziness, tingling sensations, blinking, etc., at activation.

The sound detection test makes it possible to evaluate the ability of the patient to respond to the presence or absence of sounds of different frequencies: instrumental sounds (e.g. drum for low frequencies, 0.5 kHz; bell for medium frequencies, from 1 to 2 kHz; rattle for high frequencies, 4 kHz) were delivered at an intensity of 70 dB HL.

Other Psychoacoustic Tests

Electrical stimulation thresholds, were obtained using 500-ms tone bursts presented at a level that was adjusted to the lowest at which the listener reported hearing the burst on at least 3 out of 5 presentations. The results were taken as an index of electrode proximity to excitable neurons [13, 15].

Electrode selectivity was evaluated with forward masking to quantify interaction between electrodes [15] using a 250-ms masker that was presented to a middle electrode at a level that was comfortably loud. Ten milliseconds after offset of the masker, a 25-ms signal was delivered to another electrode in the same row of electrodes along the implant array. The listener heard two intervals: both contained the masker but only one, selected randomly, contained the signal. The level of the signal was adjusted adaptively according to a 3 down, 1 up rule to converge on the signal level that would produce 79% correct detection. This level was used as the masked threshold. Masking was calculated as the elevation of the signal above the quiet threshold for the same stimulus, measured in dB. Masking typically diminished as the distance was increased between the electrode that received the masker and the one that received the signal. The width of the interference was interpolated as the distance in mm between electrodes where the masking dropped by 1 dB from the peak masking level.

Amplitude modulation detection, was determined in a 2 alternative forced-choice adaptive task, and used as an indication of temporal resolution. A 400-ms unmodulated biphasic pulse train (200 μs/phase, 250 pps) was presented in one of the intervals selected at random. The other interval contained the same carrier stimulus and was sinusoidal amplitude modulated at either 10 or 20 Hz [16]. The modulation depth was adjusted adaptively to obtain the level that produced 79% correct responses. The modulation detection threshold was computed from the last 8 reversals in the adaptive procedure.

The average modulation detection threshold was computed for at least four levels of loudness ranging from very soft to very loud. There was a significant difference ($p < 0.001$) between nontumor and NF2 with amplitude modulation values of -22.7 (9.0) and -14.0 (6.1), respectively.

Speech understanding of single phonemes (vowels) and simple sentences (HINT) [17] was determined.

Average, standard deviation and statistical outcomes of the psychoacoustic and speech test results obtained in 39 patients, 25 nontumor and 14 tumor

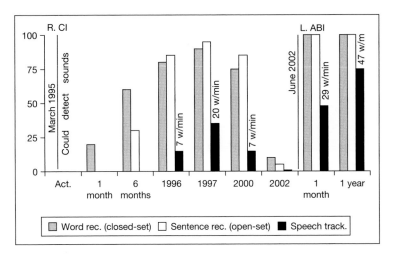

Fig. 5. Cochlear and auditory brainstem outcomes in a patient (T.L.; 26-year-old female) with cochlear bilateral ossification (for description, see text). Speech tracking is reported as arbitrary scores (65 words/min corresponding to 100%).

patients are listed in table 1. For a detailed description of the test procedures used, see Shannon and Otto [18] and Colletti and Shannon [19].

Patients Who Had Previously Received a Cochlear Implant

Four patients who had previously been fitted with cochlear implants and initially experiencing good open-set speech recognition, had over time experienced a deterioration of the performance of the device. After contralateral ABI implantation, most of these patients obtained excellent open-set speech understanding, including use of the telephone for normal conversation. An example of a patient (T.L.) with bilateral cochlear ossification that was fitted on one side with a cochlear implant and with an ABI on the other side is described in figure 5. This patient had acquired bilateral profound hearing loss from a viral infection at age 8. At age 15, she underwent tympanoplasty with mastoidectomy on the left ear to treat a cholesteatoma. At age 17, she was fitted with a cochlear implant on the right ear and reached 90% open-set sentence recognition after 2 years. Subsequently, her hearing deteriorated with dramatic reduction in sentence recognition following a progressive diffuse ossification of the left cochlea (fig. 2c). An attempt to insert a cochlear implant via a subtemporal approach was performed on August 20, 2001. At this operation, the cochlea proved to be completely filled with dense bone with no evidence of a cochlear lumen and it

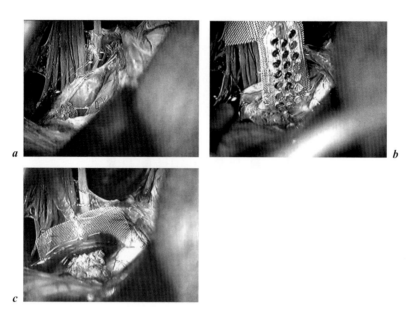

a

b

c

Fig. 6. ABI insertion into the left lateral recess using retrosigmoid approach. The cochlear nucleus is identified since it bulges in the floor of the lateral recess (*a*), and the electrode array is then completely inserted into the lateral recess (*b, c*).

was not possible to insert the array. An ABI was implanted on the left side in June 2002 (fig. 6). One month after activation of the ABI, she scored 100% at word and sentence recognition in the auditory-only mode and 29 words/min at the speech tracking test. At 1 year after receiving the ABI, she scored 47 words/min in the speech tracking test. She now uses the telephone routinely for normal conversation.

Discussion

Bilateral hearing loss from removals of bilateral vestibular schwannoma in patients with NF2 is the most common indication for rehabilitation with ABIs. While 75–85% of such patients get auditory sensations from the use of an ABI and most patients obtain environmental sound awareness and understanding of closed-set words, consonants and vowels, the results are not better than what was achieved with single-channel cochlear implants and thus significantly worse than what is presently achieved by modern multichannel cochlear implants. Significant functional auditory-alone speech recognition is the exception rather than the norm [16, 20–26] for ABIs used by NF2 patients. Combined with cues from lip-reading, 90% of patients may achieve improved sentence understanding at 6–12 months after implantation provided they receive adequate training [16, 20–26].

Recent experience has shown that patients with other causes of cochlear nerve dysfunction than tumors achieve far better results from use of ABIs and their speech discrimination is similar to that obtained with modern multichannel cochlear implants [5, 8, 19, 27]. Our experience of the performance of ABIs in nontumor patients who had various forms of cochlear nerve disorders makes us confident that many nontumor patients would benefit from the use of ABIs. In fact we believe that such patients are ideal candidates for restoration of hearing through ABI.

Patients with severe impairment of the function of the cochlear nerve, such as from aplasia or avulsion after head injury with cochlear fractures, do not benefit from cochlear implants, and it is often impossible to insert a cochlear electrode array in patients with severe abnormalities of the cochlea, such as malformations or acquired ossification. We have shown that such patients benefit from the use of an ABI [5–8] and that the benefit is similar to what would have been obtained if a modern multichannel cochlear implants could have been used.

Various degrees of hearing loss associated with cochlear ossification occur in approximately 15% of adult patients, and in 28–35% of children [28, 29]. Approximately 25% of patients with congenital sensorineural hearing loss have radiologically identifiable morphologic abnormalities of the inner ear [30]. Inner ear malformations are associated with many forms of hearing deficits [31]. Recently, Kriskovich et al. [32] used MRI and CT to study 198 individuals with congenital sensory neural hearing loss; 14 of these individuals had absence or hypoplasia of the cochlear nerve. Following severe head injury, 17–56% of patients present with variable degrees of hearing loss and in 8% there is severe or profound impairment [33, 34].

The widely held notion that the ABI yields poor rehabilitative hearing results as compared to those achieved with cochlear implants may be the main reason for not extending the use of ABIs to other patients than those who had bilateral vestibular schwannoma removed.

Naturally, operations in the posterior fossa involve certain risks, and gaining access to the foramen of Luschka and to the cochlear nuclei at the brainstem is a potentially dangerous maneuver, but, in expert hands, it has not at all increased the prevalence of complications such as cerebellar edema, ischemia or intracranial infection. The surgical procedure for ABI implantation is similar to many other surgical procedures currently used routinely in neurotology such as vestibular neurectomy to treat Ménière's disease, neurovascular decompression of cranial nerves for trigeminal neuralgia, hemifacial spasm, disabling positional vertigo, tinnitus, or spasmodic torticollis. The incidence of complications is quite negligible in this procedure, and we strongly believe that total deafness is no less incapacitating than some of the above-mentioned diseases that are treated routinely by operations that are similar to those of implantation of an electrode array in the lateral recess of the fourth ventricle.

The surgical approach for removal of vestibular schwannoma that is currently used in most otologic centers is the translabyrinthine approach. This route requires destructive surgical steps including complete mastoidectomy, labyrinthectomy, and opening of the internal auditory canal, with the risk of injuring the facial nerve. In addition, abdominal fat is needed to seal the temporal bone cavity. We prefer the retrosigmoid (retromastoid) approach because it is faster than the translabyrinthine approach; the bone area to be removed is limited and there are fewer critical structures liable to be damaged in order to reach the foramen of Luschka. The mastoid air cells are bypassed, thus preventing intracranial infection with the middle ear flora.

Attempts to improve the results of ABI include development of penetrating microelectrodes. However, none of the patients with multiple penetrating electrodes have achieved significant open set speech recognition, even after a year of implant experience. The fact that nontumor patients can achieve a high level of speech understanding with an ABI indicate that the surface array technology for ABIs is sufficient to produce excellent open-set speech understanding and that there is no need for penetrating electrodes in the CN.

The reason for the marked difference in performance between NF2 patients and patients with other causes of cochlear nerve dysfunction is not known, but several hypotheses have been presented. Unlike patients with NF2 and bilateral removals of vestibular schwannoma, patients with other causes of cochlear nerve dysfunction do not have any compression or dislocation of the brainstem and their central auditory system is likely to be fairly normal.

An alternate hypothesis, the bypass hypothesis, claims that the difference in speech understanding between cochlear implant and ABI is due to the fact the ABI bypasses or distorts the activation of specialized neural circuitry located in the CN. Cochlear implants directly stimulate the cochlear nerve and allow some of the intrinsic specialized CN circuitry to work in a relatively normal fashion, while the ABI directly stimulates the surface of the CN, simultaneously activates only some of the neural pathways that are normally activated and thereby possibly prevents activation of neurons that specialize in kinds of processing that are important for speech discrimination [Møller, this vol, pp 206–223].

The results of the use of ABIs in patients with injury to the cochlear nerve from other causes than a tumor and removal of the tumor [4, 27] who demonstrated excellent open-set speech recognition indicate that electrical stimulation of the cochlear nucleus can indeed provide speech discrimination similar to what is obtained by multichannel cochlear implants. This means that the cause of the poor performance in NF2 patients is not failure of ABIs to stimulate cochlear nucleus cells but it must have other yet unknown causes [Møller, this vol, pp 206–223].

We have shown a highly significant difference in speech recognition and in modulation detection between tumor and nontumor patients, but there were no significant differences in electrical threshold levels, electrode selectivity, the range of loudness or pitch perception evoked by the ABIs between these groups. One possible explanation for the difference in performance of ABIs in tumor and nontumor patients may be that the tumor growth and/or surgical tumor removal induce damage of a portion of the cochlear nucleus that is critical for speech recognition.

The fact that the surface array technology of the existing ABI is sufficient to produce excellent open-set speech recognition in nontumor patients indicates that the poor results in NF2 patients may be attributed to a specific disease process (or to the relative treatments) involving the cochlear nuclei and not to tonotopy mismatch.

It is puzzling why NF2 ABI patients have not been able to understand open-set speech, when their basic perceptual capabilities appear to be intact. Thus, studies have generally shown that psychophysical measures are poorly correlated with speech recognition [35, 36] with the exception of a study by Fu [16] who showed a close correlation in cochlear implant listeners between modulation detection and phoneme recognition ($r^2 = 0.97$ for consonants and $r^2 = 0.72$ for vowels). The data from the present study on ABI patients confirm Fu's [16] study and show a high correlation between modulation detection and speech recognition in patients fitted with ABIs. The difference in performance between NF2 and nontumor patients may therefore reflect a difference in the survival of a specific neuronal pathway that is critical for both modulation detection ability and speech understanding and not for electrode threshold or selectivity.

The fact that nontumor patients can achieve a high level of speech understanding with an ABI may have implications for the use of ABIs in NF2 patients, and the following changes in the surgical procedures for removal of vestibular schwannoma may be suggested. (1) Surgical removal of vestibular schwannoma in NF2 patients should be done before the tumor reaches a size so that it compresses the brainstem (tumor size <1.5 cm). (2) When tumors that are larger than 2 cm are removed, a different structure of the ascending auditory pathways may be used for electrical stimulation. The inferior colliculus may be an ideal target because it is a large auditory nucleus with a relatively simple, well-characterized tonotopic map. A recently performed inferior colliculus implant in a patient with NF2 seems to confirm that the inferior colliculus may be a suitable target for implantation [37, 38].

References

1 Shannon RV, Fayad J, Moore JK, et al: Auditory brainstem implant. II. Post-surgical issues and performance. Otolaryngol Head Neck Surg 1993;108:635–643.
2 Laszig R, Aschendorff A: Cochlear implants and electrical brainstem stimulation in sensorineural hearing loss. Opin Neurol 1999;12:41–44.
3 Otto SR, Shannon RV, Brackmann DE, et al: The multichannel auditory brainstem implant: performance in twenty patients. Otolaryngol Head Neck Surg 1998;118:291–303.
4 Colletti V, Fiorino FG, Carner M, et al: Auditory brainstem implant (ABI): new prospects in adults and children. Otolaryngol Head Neck Surg 2005;133:126–138.
5 Colletti V, Carner M, Pacini L, et al: Hearing restoration with auditory brainstem implant in three children with cochlear nerve aplasia. Otol Neurotol 2002;23:682–693.
6 Colletti V, Carner M, Colletti L, et al: Cochlear implant failure: is an auditory brainstem implant the answer? Acta Otolaryngol 2004;124:353–357.
7 Colletti V, Carner M, Colletti L, et al: Auditory brainstem implant as a salvage treatment after unsuccessful cochlear implantation. Otol Neurotol 2004:485–496.
8 Colletti V, Carner M, Colletti L, et al: Auditory brainstem implant in posttraumatic cochlear nerve avulsion. Audiol Neurootol 2004;9:247–255.
9 Skinner MW, Clark GM, et al: Evaluation of a new spectral peak coding strategy for the Nucleus 22 channel cochlear implant system. Am J Otol 1994;15(suppl 2):15–27.
10 Investigational protocol for the clinical trial of the multichannel auditory brainstem implant. Cochlear Co, 1999.
11 Psarros CE, Plant KL, Lee K, et al: Conversion from the SPEAK to the ACE strategy in children using the Nucleus 24 cochlear implant system: speech perception and speech production outcomes. Ear Hear 2002;19:18S–27S.
12 Mecklenburg DJ, Dowell R, Jenison W: The Manual of Auditory Rehabilitation. Basel, Cochlear AG, 1997.
13 Ranck J: Which elements are excited in electrical stimulation of mammalian central nervous system: a review. Brain Res 1975;98:417–440.
14 Shannon RV, Moore J, McCreery D, et al: Threshold-distance measures from electrical stimulation of human brainstem. IEEE Trans Rehabil Engin 1997;5:1–5.
15 Shannon RV: Multichannel electrical stimulation of the auditory nerve in man. II. Channel interaction. Hear Res 1983;12:1–16.
16 Fu QJ: Temporal processing and speech recognition in cochlear implant users. Neuroreport 2002;13:1635–1639.
17 Nilsson M, Soli S, Sullivan JA: Development of the hearing in noise Test for the measurement of speech reception thresholds in quiet and in noise. J Acoust Soc Am 1994;95:1085–1099.
18 Shannon RV, Otto SR: Psychophysical measures from electrical stimulation of the human cochlear nucleus. Hear Res 1990;47:159–168.
19 Colletti V, Shannon RV: Open set speech perception with auditory brainstem implant? Laryngoscope 2005;115:1974–1978.
20 Laszig R, Aschendorff A: Cochlear implants and electrical brainstem stimulation in sensorineural hearing loss. Opin Neurol 1999;12:41–44.
21 Ebinger K, Otto S, Arcaroli J, et al: Multichannel auditory brainstem implant: US clinical trial results, J Laryngol Otol 2000;114:50–53.
22 Toh EH, Luxford WM: Cochlear and brainstem implantation. Otolaryngol Clin North Am 2002;35:325–342.
23 Kanowitz SJ, Shapiro WH, Golfinos JG, Cohen NL, Roland JT Jr: Auditory brainstem implantation in patients with neurofibromatosis type 2. Laryngoscope 2004;114:2135–2146.

24 Lenarz M, Matthies C, Lesinski-Schiedat A, Frohne C, Rost U, Illg A, Battmer RD, Samii M: Auditory brainstem implant. II. Subjective assessment of functional outcome. Otol Neurotol 2002;23:694–697.
25 Nevison B, Laszig R, Sollmann WP, Lenarz T, Sterkers O, Ramsden R, Fraysse B, Manrique M, Rask-Andersen H, Garcia-Ibanez E, Colletti V, von Wallenberg E: Results from a European clinical investigation of the Nucleus multichannel auditory brainstem implant. Ear Hear 2002;23: 170–183.
26 Otto SR, Brackmann DE, Hitselberger WE, Shannon RV, Kuchta J: Multichannel auditory brainstem implant: update on performance in 61 patients. J Neurosurg 2002;96:1063–1071.
27 Colletti V, Fiorino FG, Carner M, et al: The auditory brainstem implantation: the University of Verona experience. Otolaryngol Head Neck Surg 2002;127:84–96.
28 Harnsberger HR, Dart DJ, Parkin JL, et al: Cochlear implant candidates: assessment with CT and MR imaging. Radiology 1987;164:53–57.
29 Balkany T, Gantz B, Nadol JB: Multichannel cochlear implants in partially ossified cochleas. Ann Otol Rhinol Laryngol 1998;97:3–7.
30 Jensen J: Malformations of the inner ear in deaf children. Acta Radiol 1969;286:1–97.
31 Jackler RK, Luxford WM, House WF: Congenital malformations of the inner ear: a classification based on embryogenesis. Laryngoscope 1987;97:2–14.
32 Kriskovich MD, Kehy SM, Davidson CH, et al: High resolution magnetic resonance imaging in the evaluation of pediatric sensorineural hearing loss: can it replace computed tomography? Proc 15th Annu Meet Am Soc Pediatr Otolaryngol, Orlando, May 2000, p 22.
33 Griffith MV: The incidence of auditory and vestibular concussion following minor head injury. J Laryngol Otol 1979;93:253–265.
34 Kockhar MS: Hearing loss after head injury. Ear Nose Throat J 1990;69:537–542.
35 Tyler RS, Summerfield Q, Wood SJ, Fernandez M: Psychoacoustic and phonetic temporal processing in normal and hearing-impaired listeners. J Acoust Soc Amer 1982;72:740–752.
36 Festen JM, Plomp R: Relations between auditory functions in impaired hearing. J Acoust Soc Am 1983;73:652–662.
37 Colletti V, et al: Report on the first case of successful electrical stimulation of the inferior colliculus in a patient with NF2. Proc 5th Asia Pacific Symp Cochlear Implant Relat Sci, Hong Kong, November 2005.
38 Lenarz M, Lim HH, et al: Electrophysiological assessment and validation of the auditory midbrain implant (AMI) (abstract 524). ARO Midwinter Meet, New Orleans, 2005.

Vittorio Colletti, MD
Clinica ORL, Ospedale Policlinico
Via Delle Menegone, 10
IT–37134 Verona (Italy)
Tel. +39 045 8074 275, Fax +39 045 5814 73, E-Mail vittoriocolletti@yahoo.com

Møller AR (ed): Cochlear and Brainstem Implants.
Adv Otorhinolaryngol. Basel, Karger, 2006, vol 64, pp 186–205

....

Basis of Electrical Stimulation of the Cochlea and the Cochlear Nucleus

Robert K. Shepherd [a–c], *Douglas B. McCreery* [d]

[a]The Bionic Ear Institute, [b]The Royal Victorian Eye & Ear Hospital, [c]Department of Otolaryngology, The University of Melbourne, East Melbourne, Australia; [d]Neural Engineering Laboratory, Huntington Medical Research Institutes, Pasadena, Calif., USA

Abstract

Sensorineural hearing loss is the most common form of deafness in humans. In patients with a severe-profound sensorineural hearing loss therapeutic intervention can only be achieved by direct electrical stimulation of the auditory nerve via a cochlear implant, or – in cases where a cochlear implant is not a surgical option – neurons within the central auditory pathway via an auditory brainstem implant. This paper reviews the basis of electrical stimulation of these structures with an emphasis on pathophysiology and safety.

Deafness is one of the most common neurological disorders within developed countries. For example, 3.5% of children from birth to 17 years of age experience some form of hearing impairment in the United States [1]. Significantly, hearing loss is even more common in the elderly. Sensorineural hearing loss (SNHL) is the most common form of deafness in adults and is typically associated with the loss of the sensory hair cells within the cochlea. In mammals, hair cells cannot regenerate; once lost, the hearing impairment is permanent. In patients with a severe-profound SNHL, therapeutic intervention can only be achieved by direct electrical stimulation of the residual primary auditory neurons (spiral ganglion neurons, SGNs) via a cochlear implant or neurons within the cochlear nucleus (CN) via an auditory brainstem implant (ABI). The present paper reviews the physiological and pathophysiological basis of electrical stimulation of SGNs or central auditory neurons following an SNHL.

Overview of Electrical Stimulation of the Auditory Nerve

At rest, all excitable tissue (nerve and muscle cells) exhibit a transmembrane potential of typically between -50 to $-100\,mV$ depending on cell type; i.e. the cell's intracellular environment is held at a negative potential relative to the extracellular environment and the cell membrane is polarized. The potential difference across the membrane is maintained by actively pumping ions from the cell via voltage-gated ion channels embedded within the cell membrane. As charge is delivered to a neuron via a stimulating electrode the membrane will begin to depolarize. This occurs at a single site proximal to a cathode or at two distal sites for an anode [2]. As the amount of charge delivered to a nerve fiber increases, the neural membrane undergoes further depolarization until it reaches threshold, where sodium ion channels switch from a resting to an active state, allowing intracellular sodium ions to cascade across the membrane to the extracellular environment, initiating an action potential [3]. Importantly, the subsequent propagation of the action potential along its axon and the release of neurotransmitter to initiate an action potential in postsynaptic neurons are achieved using normal physiological processes and are independent of whether or not the activity was generated using natural or artificial means [2].

As noted above, electrical stimulation of neural tissue – including the auditory nerve – is a charge-dependent process. Since charge is the product of current and time, neurons are sensitive to changes in both current amplitude and stimulus duration. Consequently, the percept of loudness in cochlear implants and ABIs can be controlled by variation in both current and pulse width [4].

Electrical stimulation of the auditory nerve using electrochemically safe biphasic current pulses (see section Electrical Stimulation of the Auditory Nerve: Safety and Efficacy below) evokes highly synchronous and deterministic discharge patterns in SGNs within a very restricted dynamic range. These response properties differ considerably from the stochastic discharge patterns observed in response to acoustic stimulation and presumably contribute to some of the perceptual differences reported between electric and acoustic hearing. Before examining the safety and efficacy of electrical stimulation of the auditory nerve, we examine the response of the cochlea to SNHL and determine what effect these changes have on the auditory nerve in deafened cochleae.

Response of the Cochlea to an SNHL

Cochlear hair cells are sensitive to many forms of pathological damage including acoustic trauma, ototoxic drugs, congenital abnormalities and aging. Following the loss of the sensory epithelium and the support cells of the organ of Corti, SGNs undergo a number of important changes that will affect the way they respond to a cochlear implant [5]. First, there is a rapid and extensive loss of the unmyelinated peripheral processes within the organ of Corti. This is followed by a more gradual degeneration of the myelinated portion of the peripheral processes within the osseous spiral lamina and of the cell bodies within Rosenthal's canal, the demyelination of surviving SGNs, and atrophy of synaptic structures in endings of the auditory nerve as they connect with the CN. The perikaryon of residual SGNs undergoes considerable shrinkage and finally the neuron undergoes cell death.

Secondary degeneration of SGNs following hair cell loss is an ongoing process, eventually resulting in small numbers of surviving neurons as has been widely reported across mammalian species (including human) following various etiologies that target the organ of Corti [5, 6]. The rate of SGN degeneration exhibits considerable variation across species. For example, human temporal bone studies typically exhibit significantly slower rates of SGN degeneration compared with studies involving experimental animals. Moreover, the degeneration rate is also dependent on etiology and severity of the pathology. Bacterial or viral labyrinthitis, for example, typically induce a more extensive pattern of neural degeneration compared with ototoxic drugs, presbyacusis or a congenital SNHL [6].

These degenerative changes to SGNs following deafness have important implications for our ability to electrically stimulate surviving neurons via a cochlear implant. The functional implications of these pathological changes will be discussed in the following section, while in the section Tropic Effects of Electrical Stimulation and Exogenous Neurotrophins we shall discuss potential techniques designed to prevent or 'rescue' SGNs from cell death following deafness.

Functional Consequences of Pathology to the Auditory Nerve

Although SGNs undergo extensive pathological changes following an SNHL, they remain capable of initiating and propagating action potentials elicited via an electrical stimulus, even in cochleae deafened for many years, with surviving neural populations of <5% of normal [5]. While the basic response properties of SGNs in deafened cochleae remain similar to those observed in normal cochleae, i.e. the cells show an increase in the probability of firing and a decrease in both response latency and the jitter in the timing of the response with increasing stimulus current, subtle changes are evident following long periods of deafness. First, loss of peripheral process and ongoing loss of SGNs result in an increase in threshold. Second, the loss of myelin will result in an increase in membrane capacitance, reducing the efficiency of a neuron initiating and propagating an action potential as evidenced by the reduction in temporal resolution [7], and an increase in refractory properties and conduction block [5] in myelin-deficient or long-term-deafened cochleae. Finally, deafness-induced changes to the synaptic structure in the endings of the auditory nerve produce alterations to synaptic transmission in the CN [8] and may contribute to the loss of temporal resolution of central auditory neurons in neonatally deafened animals [5, 9]. Importantly, these pathologically induced changes in neural response properties have the potential to degrade the functionality of cochlear implants, particularly with respect to temporal processing, while increased thresholds will have an adverse effect on implant power consumption and result in a reduction in spatial selectivity of the electrode array [10].

Electrical Stimulation of the Auditory Nerve: Safety and Efficacy

While most forms of charge delivery result in damage to surrounding tissue, nondamaging electrical stimulation can be achieved using short duration ($<300\,\mu s$/phase) charge-balanced biphasic current pulses delivered using platinum electrodes and operating – for electrodes located within the cochlea – at charge densities of $<60\,\mu C/cm^{-2}$ geom/phase [5]. These guidelines ensure that the delivery of charge to the biological environment is achieved via reversible electrochemical reactions localized to the electrode-tissue interface, minimizing the chance of releasing harmful electrochemical products into the tissue environment [11]. Contemporary cochlear implants operating using a monopolar electrode configuration would typically produce charge densities of an order of a magnitude below these levels.

Theoretically, charge-balanced biphasic current pulses should not result in the production of potentially damaging direct current, however in practice it is not possible to generate perfectly balanced stimuli. Within the cochlea, SGN loss and new bone formation as a result of tissue necrosis are observed following chronic stimulation with direct current levels greater than $0.4\,\mu A$. Protection against direct current, and the local pH changes that occur as a result of charge imbalance, can be achieved by either shorting electrodes between current pulses and/or by placing a capacitor in series with the electrode [4, 12]. One or a combination of these techniques is used to ensure complete charge recovery in contemporary cochlear implant systems.

Patient selection criteria for a cochlear implant has recently been extended from the profoundly deaf to now include severely deaf patients that receive little benefit from a conventional hearing aid. Some of these patients have relatively good hearing at low frequencies. Attempts have been made to take advantage of this residual hearing by providing both electric and acoustic stimulation in the one ear in order to provide improved speech perception [Roland and Wright, this vol, pp 11–30]. Experimental [13] and clinical studies [14, 15] have shown that hair cells apical to the electrode array can survive long-term cochlear implantation and electrical stimulation. Clinical results typically show that combined electric and acoustic stimulation to the one ear provides improved speech perception over electrical stimulation alone; this is particularly true for the perception of speech in noise [14, 15]. While promising, further research is required to optimize the electrode arrays and their insertion protocols, together with refinement of electric/acoustic speech processing strategies. Finally, long-term clinical experience will be necessary to determine whether the advantages of electric/acoustic hearing can be maintained over extended periods of time.

Due to the inherent inefficiency of the transcutaneous radiofrequency link supplying power and data to the implanted stimulator, any technique that minimizes electrical thresholds can dramatically reduce the power consumption of a cochlear implant [4], leading to the development of smaller devices and the potential for increased numbers of electrode contacts. Any change to the electrical stimulus waveform or the geometry of the electrode array may impact on power consumption and therefore implant design.

The occurrence of the second (hyperpolarizing) phase of a biphasic current pulse – while necessary for electrochemical safety – can influence auditory nerve excitability. There is a finite time (in the order of 10's of μs) between delivering a suprathreshold depolarizing charge to the neural membrane and the initiation of an action potential. Delivering a large hyperpolarizing charge within this period reduces the probability of action potential generation. Biphasic current pulses incorporating an interphase gap of the order of 50 μs or more are now typically used in cochlear implants [4] as these stimulus waveforms exhibit lower thresholds [16, 17].

There is also interest in using asymmetric biphasic, or symmetrical triphasic current pulses that are designed to achieve the necessary charge balancing between phases, but minimize the influence of the hyperpolarizing phase – thereby increasing the efficacy of the stimulus [17, 18]. Moreover, there is evidence that these waveforms provide improved spatial selectivity [10], giving rise to the possibility of an increased number of independent channels.

Monopolar and, to a lesser extent, bipolar electrode configurations are most commonly used clinically [4]. Bipolar stimulation is achieved using two electrodes located within the cochlea, and produces quite a localized pattern of excitation [19]. However, if the electrodes are not located close to SGNs, thresholds are relatively high [20] as a result of current shunting. In contrast, monopolar stimulation consists of a single electrode within the cochlea stimulated against a large surface area remote electrode located outside the cochlea. This results in a very efficient electrode configuration producing low thresholds [21] while evoking electrode-place pitch percepts consistent with the tonotopic organization of the cochlea [22]. The widespread use of monopolar electrodes clinically has increased the efficiency of cochlear implants more than any other single technique.

There is also interest in the use of tripolar and quadrupolar electrodes, particularly for the possibility of producing 'virtual' electrodes using current focusing techniques [23]. Although these electrodes are capable of producing very restrictive excitation patterns they require considerably more charge to excite SGNs compared to a monopolar electrode. The clinical application of these electrode geometries is yet to be determined and will be a trade-off between the potential advantages of increased electrode numbers versus the disadvantage of their reduced efficiency [24].

Finally, most cochlear implant systems present biphasic current pulses sequentially to one electrode at a time in order to avoid the adverse effects of channel interaction that can occur with the simultaneous stimulation of more than one electrode [25, 26; see also Loizou, this vol, pp 109–143], although some devices can implement a simultaneous stimulation paradigm.

Trophic Effects of Electrical Stimulation and Exogenous Neurotrophins

Auditory neurons exhibit significant reductions in both driven and spontaneous activity following an SNHL such that these neurons rarely undergo depolarization. However, neural activity is known to play an important role in SGN survival; depolarization is sufficient to maintain SGN survival in vitro without the addition of neurotrophic factors by elevating intracellular calcium levels and cascading several intracellular signaling pathways [27].

A number of in vivo studies have described significant increases in SGN survival in ototoxically deafened animals following chronic electrical stimulation of the auditory nerve when compared with nonstimulated control cochleae [review: 5, 28]. The majority of these studies described modest but significant increases in neural survival associated with chronic electrical stimulation. In contrast, several studies have reported no evidence of chronic electrical stimulation providing a trophic influence on SGNs [5, 28]. In sum, it would appear that the trophic influence of chronic electrical stimulation on deafened SGNs is, at best, relatively small.

There is agreement, however, that chronic electrical stimulation in deafened ears results in morphological changes to SGNs. For example, there is a small but significant increase in the soma area of SGNs in deafened chronically stimulated cochleae compared with deafened controls [29]. This increase in soma area presumably reflects an increase in biosynthetic activity within the SGN soma following reactivation via an electrical stimulus, and reflects earlier reports describing increased soma area in second-order neurons of the ventral CN following chronic electrical stimulation in deafened animals [30].

Significantly, chronic stimulation of the auditory nerve in deafened animals has also been shown to restore normal synaptic structure in endings of the auditory nerve that atrophy following deafness as a result of loss of activity [31]. Restoration of these synapses may contribute to the improved temporal resolution of auditory midbrain neurons following chronic electrical stimulation [32].

Recently, there has been considerable interest in the application of exogenous growth factors such as neurotrophins to promote SGN survival following deafness. A number of growth factor families have been shown to play important roles in the development, maintenance and protection against injury of SGNs [33]. Both presynaptic hair cells and postsynaptic neurons within the CN are necessary for SGN survival through the release of endogenous neurotrophins [34]. These neurotrophins include both brain-derived neurotrophic factor and neurotrophin-3; with receptors for both of these neurotrophins expressed on SGNs [34]. Importantly, survival of SGNs in the absence of hair cells has been promoted by exogenous brain-derived neurotrophic factor or neurotrophin-3 in vivo [review: 35]. In contrast to the relatively modest survival effects of electrical stimulation, exogenous delivery of neurotrophins typically results in highly significant survival effects on SGNs if applied to the cochlea soon after deafening. Importantly, this work also showed a functional advantage in the form of significantly reduced electrically-evoked auditory brainstem response thresholds in ears treated with neurotrophins [36, 37].

While these results are promising, from a clinical perspective further research is necessary before neurotrophins can be combined with cochlear implants. Rescue of SGNs is only effective via a continuous delivery of neurotrophins [38], therefore the long-term safety and efficacy of neurotrophin delivery to the cochlea must be clearly established.

Overview of Electrical Stimulation of the Auditory Brainstem

While cochlear implants have restored hearing to tens of thousands of patients with a severe-profound SNHL, those who lack a functional auditory nerve cannot benefit from these devices. However, a prosthesis utilizing an electrode array implanted adjacent to the CN can restore some hearing. Worldwide, several hundred patients have received ABIs; at the House Ear Clinic/House Ear Institute in Los Angeles, Calif., USA, more than 200 patients afflicted with type

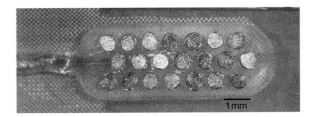

Fig. 1. An array of 21 platinum disc electrodes used in the present version of the ABI manufactured by Cochlear Ltd. The platinum electrodes are mounted on a carrier of silicone elastomer.

2 neurofibromatosis (NF2) have received ABIs [39–42]. NF2 occurs in about one in 40,000 live births [43], and these patients typically develop life-threatening vestibular schwannoma on the 8th nerve, with a high probability that the tumors will occur bilaterally [44]. The usual outcome is total destruction of the auditory and vestibular components of both 8th nerves, either by the invasive tumor itself, or during its surgical resection. After the tumor has been removed surgically, the ABI's electrode array is placed within the lateral recess of the 4th ventricle. Figure 1 shows the present version of the electrode array, which includes 21 disk-shaped platinum electrodes, each 0.7 mm in diameter, spaced at intervals of 1 mm and embedded in a matrix of silicone elastomer.

Functional Anatomy of the CN

The CN complex is located on the dorsolateral surface of the brainstem at the junction of the medulla and the pons. In humans, the dorsal nucleus curves over the inferior cerebellar peduncle. The ventral CN lies partly beneath the lateral portion of the dorsal CN and beneath the pontobulbar body, spanning ~3 mm along its dorsoventral and rostrocaudal dimensions. The cytoarchitecture of the ventral CN complex is quite similar in most mammalian species, although the proportions of the different cell types are somewhat variable across species [45]. Figure 2 depicts the human CN complex and that of the domestic cat. The ventral nucleus consists of a rostral area of spherical cells, a caudal region containing octopus cells, and a central region where globular cells, a heterogeneous population of multipolar cells, and small cells are intermixed [45, 46]. In humans, the dorsal nucleus lies within the lateral recess of the 4th ventricle, while the ventral nucleus extends to the foramen of Luschka.

In all species in which it has been investigated, a cochleotopic (tonotopic) sequence of terminations of auditory nerve axons has been demonstrated [47–51]. The axonal branching pattern of the ventral CN appears to be very similar in cats

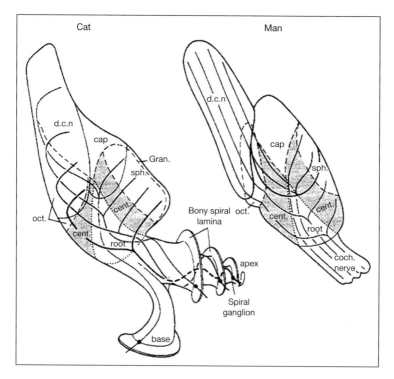

Fig. 2. A diagrammatic representation of the human and feline CN complexes, seen in lateral views. The portion of the central nucleus containing the stellate/multipolar cells is stippled (reprinted from Moore and Osen, 1979 [46], by permission of the publisher).

and humans. Figure 3 shows a histologic section through the human ventral CN. In humans, the posterior segment of the central nucleus lies within 1 mm of the free surface of the brainstem, beneath the pontobulbar body and the glial-pia overlayer. This portion of the central nucleus, the homologue of the feline posteroventral CN, contains the multipolar cells which project directly to the inferior colliculus [46], and as such are likely to be one of the neuronal population that mediates monaural hearing. In humans, damage to the ventral acoustic stria of the trapezoid body, which contains afferent axons from the ventral nucleus, produces severe hearing loss and severe impairment of speech perception [52].

Electrical Stimulation of the CN

As with any neural prosthesis, an ABI must induce action potentials in the requisite population of neurons, or in their axons. For ABI patients from the

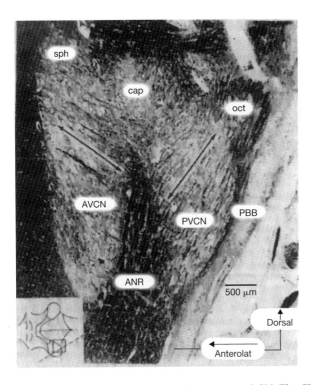

Fig. 3. A section through the human ventral CN. The CN has been embedded in celloidin and sectioned along the long axis of the nucleus in a rotated sagittal plane. In this plane, the anterior end of the nucleus is rotated laterally by ~30°, as shown in the inset drawing in the horizontal plane. The section has been stained with cresyl violet and iron hematoxylin to demonstrate both cells and myelinated axons. The superficial posterior surface of the nucleus is covered by the pontobulbar body (PBB). Individual fibers of the auditory nerve bifurcate within the nerve root (ANR). The direction of the diverging terminal branches within the anteroventral and posteroventral divisions of the nucleus (AVCN, PVCN) is indicated by arrows. Areas containing spherical cells (sph), octopus cells (oct) and the small cell cap (cap) are indicated. Modified from McCreery et al. [70].

House Ear Clinic, threshold charge for auditory percepts ranges from less than 10 nC/phase (each phase of the stimulus pulse pair) to more than 200 nC/phase, using charge-balanced pulses of 300 μs in duration [39, 53]. The reason for the large variability between patients is unclear, but since the threshold for a particular patient tends to remain quite stable over time, the variability may reflect differences in the placement of the electrode array and possibly different amounts of damage to the CN inflicted by the disease process (NF2).

The response of neurons in the central nervous system (CNS) to electrical stimulation usually is characterized in terms of their current distant constant (k) and their membrane time constant. In this respect, neurons of the human CN that mediate auditory percepts appear to be quite typical of other neurons of the mammalian CNS. The Hill equation describes the relationship between threshold stimulus current (I), stimulus charge per phase (Q), stimulus pulse duration (t), and the membrane time constant (J): $Q = It/(1 - e^{-t/J})$. The time constant for the neuronal elements in the human CN that mediate auditory percepts near threshold is 1 ms or less [39, 54, 55]. For comparison, the time constants of myelinated axons in the mammalian CNS range from ~50 to 100 μs [56], and from ~200 μs to 10 ms for cell bodies and their dendrites [57–59]. The rather long time constant for the auditory percepts produced by stimulating the human CN suggests that at near threshold, the electrical stimulus activates cell bodies or their dendrites, or the initial segment of the axon proximal to the cell body [60], rather than the axons at a site distal to their soma.

Most studies indicate that the amplitude of the stimulus current (I) required to excite neurons in the CNS varies as the square of the distance between a small (point source) electrode and the neuron; $I = kd^2$. Since current density (i) in tissue decreases as the square of distance (d) from a point source electrode, the current-distance relation can be expressed in terms of the threshold current density; $k = 4\pi i$ [61]. As noted above, the threshold current for auditory percepts varies greatly for different users of the ABI, but for some patients the threshold is less than 10 nC/phase, or about 33 μA for a pulse duration of 300 μs [53]. The platinum electrodes of the array shown in figure 1 are ~0.7 mm in diameter (0.4 mm²), giving an averaged current density at the surface of the electrode at a threshold of ~80 μA/mm². As illustrated in figure 3, neurons of the human ventral CN are at least 0.5 mm beneath the free surface of the brainstem, under the pontobulbar body, where the current density would be lower than at the surface of the electrode, and thus less than 80 μA/mm² for the patients with the lowest thresholds for auditory percepts. For these patients, $k < 4\pi 80$ μA/mm² = 1,000 μA/mm², which is quite typical of neurons of the mammalian CNS where k ranges from ~250 to 4,000 μA/mm² [61].

Penetrating Microelectrodes

An array of 'macroelectrodes' of the type shown in figure 1, which resides on the surface of the brainstem, can activate neurons throughout much of the underlying CN. However, the current from these relatively large electrodes must spread quite broadly, providing only limited access to the spatial organization of the underlying nucleus, including its tonotopic organization [42]. In contrast, microelectrodes that penetrate into the tissue can excite highly localized

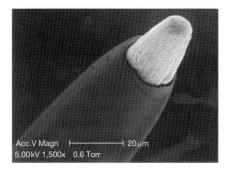

Acc.V Magn   ├─────────────┤ 20 μm
5.00kV 1,500x 0.6 Torr

Fig. 4. A scanning electron micrograph of an activated iridium microelectrode. The insulation (Parylene-C) has been removed for ~2,000 μm² at the tip.

populations of neurons and in principle should allow more precise and orderly access to the nucleus' tonotopic organization. Thus, a neural prosthesis that employs both macro- and microelectrodes might provide improved hearing. The feasibility of microstimulation within the CN has been investigated using animal models in several laboratories [62–69]. McCreery et al. [70] applied microstimulation at various locations along the dorsoventral axis of the feline posteroventral CN while recording multiunit activity and local field potentials at 20 or more locations along the tonotopic axis of the central nucleus of the contralateral inferior colliculus. The study showed that microstimulation within the posteroventral CN can access the tonotopic organization of the nucleus in an orderly manner. This can be attributed not only to the highly localized nature of the microstimulation but also to the trajectory of the axons of the afferent projections from the feline CN. In the cat, the afferent axons traverse medially and slightly ventrally across the nucleus, approximately parallel to the isofrequency lamina, as defined by the terminations of auditory nerve fibers. The same arrangement appears to be present in humans [45, 46]. Were this not the case, the electrodes would tend to excite axons from multiple isofrequency lamina, rendering it much more difficult to access the nucleus' tonotopic organization in an orderly manner. As could be expected, the threshold for the induction of neuronal activity by the microstimulation is very low. McCreery et al. [69, 68, 70] implanted iridium microelectrodes of the type shown in figure 4 into the feline ventral CN. The field potentials induced by the intranuclear microstimulation were recorded via electrodes implanted chronically over the contralateral inferior colliculus. The thresholds of the responses evoked by 150 μs/phase charge-balanced pulses ranged from slightly less than 5 μA to 10 μA (0.75–1.5 nC/phase). In one cat with electrodes implanted for 7 years, the response threshold was 5 ± 1 μA for the first 5 years, increasing to about 7 μA by the end of the 7th year [69]. In other cats, implanted for periods of up to 20 months, response thresholds were 5–7 μA (0.75–1 nC/phase) [68].

Recently, clinical trials have begun of a hybrid ABI, which includes the surface array depicted in figure 1 and also an array of 8 activated iridium microelectrodes. In one recipient, 5 of the penetrating microelectrodes induced auditory percepts, which were described as tones of various pitches. The thresholds for the percepts range from ~0.8 to 2 nC/phase; in contrast, the threshold for auditory percepts induced by the macroelectrodes of the surface array range from 10 to 100 nC/phase; the higher values corresponded to the more medial electrodes, which presumably were not directly over the ventral CN [71].

Safety of Macro- and Microstimulation of the CN

Certainly, one of the requirements for any neural prosthesis must be the ability to activate the requisite neurons without causing injury to the neurons or to other tissue elements. There are several mechanisms by which electrical stimulation might inflict tissue injury [see section Electrical Stimulation of the Auditory Nerve: Safety and Efficacy above and reviewed in 72]. The propensity for stimulation-induced neural injury is determined by all of the stimulus parameters, including charge density and charge per phase [68]. As noted above, a stimulus waveform typically consists of a pair of current pulses of opposite polarity in which the charge delivered by each pulse (Q), is equal. The 'geometric' charge density is defined as the charge per phase divided by the electrode's 'geometric' surface area ($4Q/\pi D^2$ for a disc electrode of diameter D). It is generally accepted that the stimulus charge density should not exceed that for which the processes that mediate injection of significant charge into the tissue are completely reversible. This criterion does not guarantee that stimulation-induced injury will not occur [73], but it does minimize the risk of generating toxic products, including the large pH changes which are potentially injurious [74]. Polished platinum disk electrodes of the type used in the ABI array shown in figure 1 can support a charge density of $\sim 100\ \mu C/cm^2$ of geometric surface area [75]. This value is considerably less than the $400–500\ \mu C/cm^2$ determined by Brummer and Turner [76], which is often cited as the 'safe' limit for platinum and platinum-iridium alloys. However, the charge injection limit determined by Brummer and Turner requires that the electrodes be returned to a nonequilibrium potential between pulses, which is not the case with the implantable stimulators now in clinical use. Some of the patients fitted with the ABI require up to 300 nC/phase in order for the auditory percepts to reach the level of maximum comfortable loudness, which corresponds to a geometric charge density of 75 $\mu C/cm^2$ for the arrays shown in figure 1. This is near, but does not exceed, the maximum value recommended for smooth platinum. At least in the cat's cerebral cortex, charge per phase and charge density interact to determine the propensity for tissue damage. The analogous study has not been conducted for macroelectrodes implanted over the CN, but in the cerebral cortex, the combination of 75 μC/cm^2 and 300 nC/phase would not be expected to be injurious [73]. This is consistent with the observation that the stimulus amplitude for threshold and maximum comfortable loudness levels for the ABI users are quite stable for many years [40, 42].

Safety of Penetrating Microelectrodes

There is a risk of mechanical tissue damage using penetrating microelectrodes both during their insertion through the highly vascular brain tissue, and during long-term implantation in the brain. There also is the opportunity for injury via electrical stimulation per se. Due to the small geometric surface areas of these electrodes (typically 1,000–5,000 μm^2), the stimulus charge density at the electrode surface typically exceeds that recommended for chronic stimulation with platinum or platinum alloys. However, activated (oxidized) iridium electrodes of the type depicted in figure 4 support electrochemical processes not shared by platinum or its alloys, which greatly increase their safe charge injection capacity [77, 78].

Niparko et al. [63] reported that 20 h of intermittent stimulation with chronically implanted microelectrodes in the guinea pig CN, at stimulation intensities of 150 and 200 μA (~600 and 800 μC/cm^2 phase) produced significant tissue response at the site of the electrode tip, with necrosis, cell loss, and reactive cells present, but the neuronal damage was observed to occur at an intensity far greater than that required for eliciting an electrophysiologic response. McCreery et al. [65, 66, 68] investigated the safety of microstimulation in the feline ventral CN with chronically implanted iridium microelectrodes similar to those shown in figure 4. Figure 5 shows tissue surrounding an iridium microelectrode implanted chronically in the ventral CN and stimulated continuously for 8 h at 500 Hz using a charge per phase of 8 nC (400 μC/cm^2). The spongiform changes in the neuropil surrounding the tip site are vacuolations of the myelinated axons [66]. In contrast, the neuronal cell bodies embedded in the damaged neuropil appear quite normal. The mechanisms responsible for the injury to the myelinated axons have not been determined with certainty, but they do resemble the spongiform vacuoles seen in the ventral CN of gerbils exposed to noise [79], suggesting that the damage is related to overstimulation.

The threshold for the injury depicted in figure 5 is 3–4 nC/phase (150–200 μC/cm^2) at a pulse rate of 500 Hz [66], and was not significantly lower when the duration of the stimulation was extended to 10–21 days [68]. However, the propensity for stimulation-induced damage to the myelinated axons of peripheral

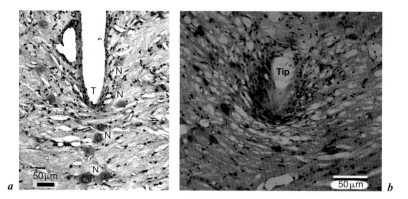

Fig. 5. *a* A histologic section through the tip site of an activated iridium microelectrode implanted chronically in a cat's CN and pulsed continuously for 8 h at 3 nC/phase, 150 µC/cm², at a rate of 500 Hz. N = Cell bodies of CN neurons. *b* The site of an electrode pulsed for 8 h at 8 nC/phase, 400 µC/cm², and 500 Hz. The spongiform appearance of the surrounding neuropil is due to vacuolations of the myelinated axons.

nerves is strongly and positively correlated with stimulus pulse rate [80]. Thus in a recent study using chronically implanted iridium microelectrodes with somewhat larger surface areas (5,000 µm²), we found that no tissue damage was induced by 8 h of stimulation at 8 nC/phase (160 µC/cm²) at a pulse rate of 250 Hz [71]. Neurons within 100 µm of the pulsed and unpulsed (control) microelectrode tips appear undamaged, and there was no evidence of the vacuoles, which were the cardinal feature of stimulation-induced injury seen in the early study, in which the pulse rate was higher.

Future Prospects of ABIs

Certainly, a number of challenging problems must be surmounted in the future development of ABIs. By their nature, these devices bypass part of the neuronal circuitry of the lower auditory system that encodes the various features of speech and environmental sounds, and there remains much uncertainty as to how features of the acoustic stimulus should be encoded into the electrical stimulation. Microelectrodes offer the opportunity to access the functions of the lower auditory systems that are spatially segregated, but even with high-density microelectrodes it will be difficult to reintroduce features of the auditory environment that are encoded by different, but intermixed neuronal populations. These issues notwithstanding, the existence of patients with severe hearing loss who cannot benefit from cochlear implants provide ample incentive to continue the development of ABIs. Significantly, recent studies [53, 81] have described ABI patients with deafness of etiologies other than NF2, some of whom demonstrated open-set speech recognition [Colletti, this vol, pp 167–185]. It is not clear why patients whose deafness is due to causes other than vestibular schwannoma tend to perform much better than the tumor patients, but these results demonstrate that the indications for ABIs could be expanded beyond NF2, to include patients with cochlear nerve aplasia or avulsion, cochlear ossification and certain traumatic injuries. There is also the hope that an advanced ABI could circumvent some of the limitations of cochlear implants. For example, multichannel cochlear implants do not allow access to auditory nerve fibers representing the lowest acoustic frequencies, while access to the low-frequency regions of the CN using penetrating microelectrodes should, in principle, present no particular difficulties.

General Conclusions

Both cochlear implants and ABIs provide severe-profoundly deaf patients with important auditory cues necessary for speech perception. Although stimulating different target neurons within the auditory pathway, both prostheses initiate depolarization using well-described biophysical principles. Once an action potential is initiated, its propagation is achieved via normal physiological processes.

Like all neural prostheses, these devices operate using electrochemically safe design parameters including: the use of noble metal electrodes (typically platinum and/or iridium); short duration charge balanced biphasic current pulses operating at charge densities shown to be safe for that application (this limitation has implications for the design and size of the stimulating electrodes used), and the use of charge recovery techniques such as electrode shorting and/or capacitive coupling to ensure that no direct current is generated.

There are also important differences between electrical stimulation of the auditory nerve and the CN that must be considered. For example, the auditory nerve undergoes gradual degeneration following loss of the sensory hair cells; CN neurons atrophy but do not normally degenerate. An emphasis in cochlear implant research is the development of techniques designed to rescue SGNs from degeneration, including the potential application of exogenous neurotrophins. The stimulation of different target sites with the auditory pathway carries with it different electrode designs; the longitudinal cochlear implant electrode array typically lies within the bony scala tympani, a small distance from the SGNs, while ABI electrodes are placed on, or within, the CN complex.

Each electrode design has its own issues of safety and efficacy that continue to be addressed in ongoing research. Because ABIs bypass part of the neuronal circuitry that encodes speech and environmental sounds, speech processing strategies used with these devices should not necessarily mirror the processing strategies used in cochlear implants. Finally, while to date nearly all ABIs have been used in a small population of patients with a specific etiology (NF2), recent clinical results suggest that the indications for an ABI could be expanded to include patients with etiologies such as cochlear nerve aplasia, severe cochlear ossification and certain traumatic injuries.

Acknowledgements

We wish to acknowledge the following funding bodies that helped make this work possible. The studies conducted at the Bionic Ear Institute were funded by the Wagstaff Fellowship, Royal Victorian Eye & Ear Hospital and NIDCD Contract N01-DC-3-1005, while studies conducted at the Huntington Medical Research Institutes were supported in part by NIDCD contracts N01-DC-1-2105 and N01-DC-4-0005. We also acknowledge our colleagues who have provided great support and intellectual stimulation, and Dr. Robert Shannon for his helpful suggestions during the preparation of the manuscript.

References

1   Boyle CA, Decoufle P, Yeargin-Allsopp M: Prevalence and health impact of developmental disabilities in US children. Pediatrics 1994;93:399–403.
2   Grill WM: Electrical stimulation of the peripheral nervous system: biophysics and excitation properties; in Horch KW, Dhillon GS (eds): Neuroprosthetics: Theory and Practice. Singapore, World Scientific, 2004, pp 319–341.
3   Hodgkin AL, Huxley AF, Katz B: Measurement of current-voltage relations in the membrane of the giant axon of Loligo. J Physiol 1952; pp 116:424–448.
4   Seligman PM, Shepherd RK: Cochlear Implants; in Horch KW, Dhillon G (eds): Neuroprosthetics: Theory and practice. Singapore, World Scientific Publishing, 2004; pp 878–904.
5   Shepherd RK, Meltzer NE, Fallon JB, Ryugo DK: Consequences of deafness and electrical stimulation on the peripheral and central auditory system; in Waltzman SB, Roland TJ (eds): Cochlear Implants. New York, Thieme Medical Publishers, Inc, in press.
6   Nadol JB Jr, Young YS, Glynn RJ: Survival of spiral ganglion cells in profound sensorineural hearing loss: implications for cochlear implantation. Ann Otol Rhinol Laryngol 1989;98:411–416.
7   Zhou R, Abbas PJ, Assouline JG: Electrically evoked auditory brainstem response in peripherally myelin-deficient mice. Hear Res 1995;88:98–106.
8   Oleskevich S, Walmsley B: Synaptic transmission in the auditory brainstem of normal and congenitally deaf mice. J Physiol 2002;540:447–455.
9   Kral A, Tillein J, Heid S, Hartmann R, Klinke R: Postnatal cortical development in congenital auditory deprivation. Cereb Cortex 2005;15:552–562.
10   Frijns JH, de Snoo SL, ten Kate JH: Spatial selectivity in a rotationally symmetric model of the electrically stimulated cochlea. Hear Res 1996;95:33–48.
11   Brummer SB, Turner MJ: Electrochemical considerations for safe electrical stimulation of the nervous system with platinum electrodes. IEEE Trans Biomed Eng 1977;24:59–63.

12 Huang CQ, Shepherd RK, Carter PM, Seligman PM, Tabor B: Electrical stimulation of the auditory nerve: direct current measurement in vivo. IEEE Trans Biomed Eng 1999;46:461–470.

13 Xu J, Shepherd RK, Millard RE, Clark GM: Chronic electrical stimulation of the auditory nerve at high stimulus rates: a physiological and histopathological study. Hear Res 1997;105:1–29.

14 Gantz BJ, Turner C, Gfeller KE, Lowder MW: Preservation of hearing in cochlear implant surgery: advantages of combined electrical and acoustical speech processing. Laryngoscope 2005;115: 796–802.

15 Kiefer J, Pok M, Adunka O, et al: Combined electric and acoustic stimulation of the auditory system: results of a clinical study. Audiol Neurootol 2005;10:134–144.

16 Carlyon RP, van Wieringen A, Deeks JM, Long CJ, Lyzenga J, Wouters J: Effect of inter-phase gap on the sensitivity of cochlear implant users to electrical stimulation. Hear Res 2005;205:210–224.

17 Shepherd RK, Javel E: Electrical stimulation of the auditory nerve: II. Effect of stimulus wave-shape on single fibre response properties. Hear Res 1999;130:171–188.

18 Coste RL, Pfingst BE: Stimulus features affecting psychophysical detection thresholds for electrical stimulation of the cochlea. III. Pulse polarity. J Acoust Soc Am 1996;99:3099–3108.

19 van den Honert C, Stypulkowski PH: Single fiber mapping of spatial excitation patterns in the electrically stimulated auditory nerve. Hear Res 1987;29:195–206.

20 Shepherd RK, Hatsushika S, Clark GM: Electrical stimulation of the auditory nerve: the effect of electrode position on neural excitation. Hear Res 1993;66:108–120.

21 Miller CA, Robinson BK, Rubinstein JT, Abbas PJ, Runge-Samuelson CL: Auditory nerve responses to monophasic and biphasic electric stimuli. Hear Res 2001;151:79–94.

22 Eddington DK, Dobelle WH, Brackmann DE, Mladejovsky MG, Parkin JL: Auditory prostheses research with multiple channel intracochlear stimulation in man. Ann Otol Rhinol Laryngol 1978;87:1–39.

23 Jolly CN, Spelman FA, Clopton BM: Quadrupolar stimulation for Cochlear prostheses: modeling and experimental data. IEEE Trans Biomed Eng 1996;43:857–865.

24 Mens LH, Berenstein CK: Speech perception with mono- and quadrupolar electrode configurations: a crossover study. Otol Neurotol 2005;26:957–964.

25 White MW, Merzenich MM, Gardi JN: Multichannel cochlear implants. Channel interactions and processor design. Arch Otolaryngol 1984;110:493–501.

26 Shannon RV: Multichannel electrical stimulation of the auditory nerve in man. II. Channel interaction. Hear Res 1983;12:1–16.

27 Hegarty JL, Kay AR, Green SH: Trophic support of cultured spiral ganglion neurons by depolarization exceeds and is additive with that by neurotrophins or cAMP and requires elevation of $(Ca^{2+})i$ within a set range. J Neurosci 1997;17:1959–1970.

28 Miller AL: Effects of chronic stimulation on auditory nerve survival in ototoxically deafened animals. Hear Res 2001;151:1–14.

29 Leake PA, Hradek GT, Snyder RL: Chronic electrical stimulation by a cochlear implant promotes survival of spiral ganglion neurons after neonatal deafness. J Comp Neurol 1999;412: 543–562.

30 Matsushima JI, Shepherd RK, Seldon HL, Xu SA, Clark GM: Electrical stimulation of the auditory nerve in deaf kittens: effects on cochlear nucleus morphology. Hear Res 1991;56:133–142.

31 Ryugo DK, Kretzmer EA, Niparko JK: Restoration of auditory nerve synapses in cats by cochlear implants. Science 2005;310:1490–1492.

32 Vollmer M, Leake PA, Beitel RE, Rebscher SJ, Snyder RL: Degradation of temporal resolution in the auditory midbrain after prolonged deafness is reversed by electrical stimulation of the cochlea. J Neurophysiol 2005;93:3339–3355.

33 Fritzsch B, Pirvola U, Ylikoski J: Making and breaking the innervation of the ear: neurotrophic support during ear development and its clinical implications. Cell Tissue Res 1999;295:369–82.

34 Ylikoski J, Pirvola U, Moshnyakov M, Palgi J, Arumae U, Saarma M: Expression patterns of neurotrophin and their receptor mRNAs in the rat inner ear. Hear Res 1993;65:69–78.

35 Gillespie LN, Shepherd RK: Clinical application of neurotrophic factors: the potential for primary auditory neuron protection. Eur J Neurosci 2005;22:2123–2133.

36 Shinohara T, Bredberg G, Ulfendahl M, et al: Neurotrophic factor intervention restores auditory function in deafened animals. Proc Natl Acad Sci USA 2002;99:1657–1660.

37 Shepherd RK, Coco A, Epp SB, Crook JM: Chronic depolarization enhances the trophic effects of brain-derived neurotrophic factor in rescuing auditory neurons following a sensorineural hearing loss. J Comp Neurol 2005;486:145–158.

38 Gillespie LN, Clark GM, Bartlett PF, Marzella PL: BDNF-induced survival of auditory neurons in vivo: Cessation of treatment leads to an accelerated loss of survival effects. J Neurosci Res 2003;71:785–790.

39 Shannon RV, Otto SR: Psychophysical measures from electrical stimulation of the human cochlear nucleus. Hear Res 1990;47:159–168.

40 Otto SR, Brackmann DE, Hitselberger WE, Shannon RV, Kuchta J: Multichannel auditory brainstem implant: update on performance in 61 patients. J Neurosurg 2002;96:1063–1071.

41 Schwartz MS, Otto SR, Brackmann DE, Hitselberger WE, Shannon RV: Use of a multichannel auditory brainstem implant for neurofibromatosis type 2. Stereotact Funct Neurosurg 2003;81: 110–114.

42 Kuchta J, Otto SR, Shannon RV, Hitselberger WE, Brackmann DE: The multichannel auditory brainstem implant: how many electrodes make sense? J Neurosurg 2004;100:16–23.

43 Evans DG, Huson SM, Donnai D, et al: A genetic study of type 2 neurofibromatosis in the United Kingdom. I. Prevalence, mutation rate, fitness, and confirmation of maternal transmission effect on severity. J Med Genet 1992;29:841–846.

44 Evans DG, Lye R, Neary W, et al: Probability of bilateral disease in people presenting with a unilateral vestibular schwannoma. J Neurol Neurosurg Psychiatry 1999;66:764–767.

45 Moore JK: The human auditory brain stem: a comparative view. Hear Res 1987;29:1–32.

46 Moore JK, Osen KK: The cochlear nuclei in man. Am J Anat 1979;154:393–418.

47 Bourk TR, Mielcarz JP, Norris BE: Tonotopic organization of the anteroventral cochlear nucleus of the cat. Hear Res 1981;4:215–241.

48 Fekete DM, Rouiller EM, Liberman MC, Ryugo DK: The central projections of intracellularly labeled auditory nerve fibers in cats. J Comp Neurol 1984;229:432–450.

49 Snyder RL, Leake PA, Hradek GT: Quantitative analysis of spiral ganglion projections to the cat cochlear nucleus. J Comp Neurol 1997;379:133–149.

50 Powell TBS, Cowen WM: An experimental study of the projection of the Cochlear. J Anat 1962;96: 269–284.

51 Sando I: The anatomical relationships of the cochlear nerve fibers. Acta Oto Laryngol 1965;59: 417–435.

52 Egan CA, Davies L, Halmagyi GM: Bilateral total deafness due to pontine haematoma. J Neurol Neurosurg Psychiatry 1996;61:628–631.

53 Colletti V, Shannon RV: Open set speech perception with auditory brainstem implant? Laryngoscope 2005;115:1974–1978.

54 Shannon RV: Threshold functions for electrical stimulation of the human cochlear nucleus. Hear Res 1989;40:173–177.

55 Shannon RV, Moore JK, McCreery DB, Portillo F: Threshold-distance measures from electrical stimulation of human brainstem. IEEE Trans Rehabil Eng 1997;5:70–74.

56 Jankowska E, Roberts SJ: An electrophysiological demonstration of the axonal projections of single spinal neurons in the cat. J Physiol 1972;222:597–622.

57 Stoney SD, Thompson WD, Asanuma H: Excitation of pyramidal tract cells by intracortical microstimulation: effective extent of stimulating current. J Neurophysiol 1968;31:659–669.

58 Lux HD, Pollen DA: Electrical constants of neurons in the motor cortex of cats. J Neurophysiol 1966;20:207–220.

59 Nelson PG, Lux HD: Some electrical measurements of neuronal parameters. Biophysics J 1970;10:55–73.

60 McIntyre CC, Grill WM: Excitation of central nervous system neurons by nonuniform electric fields. Biophys J 1999;76:878–888.

61 Tehovnik EJ: Electrical stimulation of neural tissue to evoke behavioral responses. J Neurosci Methods 1996;65:1–17.

62 Evans DE, Niparko JK, Miller JM, Jyung RW, Anderson DJ: Multiple-channel stimulation of the cochlear nucleus. Otolaryngol Head Neck Surg 1989;101:651–657.

63   Niparko JK, Altschuler RA, Xue XL, Wiler JA, Anderson DJ: Surgical implantation and biocompatibility of central nervous system auditory prostheses. Ann Otol Rhinol Laryngol 1989;98: 965–970.

64   Liu X, McPhee G, Seldon HL, Clark GM: Histological and physiological effects of the central auditory prosthesis: surface versus penetrating electrodes. Hear Res 1997;114:264–274.

65   McCreery DB, Yuen TG, Agnew WF, Bullara LA: Stimulation with chronically implanted microelectrodes in the cochlear nucleus of the cat: histologic and physiologic effects. Hear Res 1992;62:42–56.

66   McCreery DB, Yuen TG, Agnew WF, Bullara LA: Stimulus parameters affecting tissue injury during microstimulation in the cochlear nucleus of the cat. Hear Res 1994;77:105–115.

67   McCreery DB, Yuen TG, Agnew WF, Bullara LA: A characterization of the effects on neuronal excitability due to prolonged microstimulation with chronically implanted microelectrodes. IEEE Trans Biomed Eng 1997;44:931–939.

68   McCreery DB, Yuen TG, Bullara LA: Chronic microstimulation in the feline ventral cochlear nucleus: physiologic and histologic effects. Hear Res 2000;149:223–238.

69   McCreery DB, Yuen TGH, Bullara LA: Physiologic and Histologic effects of prolonged microstimulation in the feline ventral cochlear nucleus. In; 2001; Conference on Implantable Auditory Prostheses, Asilomar CA (Abstract); 2001.

70   McCreery DB, Shannon RV, Moore JK, Chatterjee M: Accessing the tonotopic organization of the ventral cochlear nucleus by intranuclear microstimulation. IEEE Trans Rehabil Eng 1998;6: 391–399.

71   McCreery DB, Lossinsky AS, Shannon RV, Sr.R O: A cochlear nucleus auditory prosthesis based on microstimulation (Contract # N01-DC-4-0005 NIDCD, from the National Institutes of Health, USA). Quarterly progress report # 3 2005.

72   McCreery D: Tissue reaction to electrodes: The problem of safe and effective stimulation of neural tissue; in Horch KW, Dhillon GS (eds): Neural Prosthesis: Theory and Practice: World Scientific Publishing, River Edge, NJ, 2004, pp 592–607.

73   McCreery DB, Agnew WF, Yuen TG, Bullara L: Charge density and charge per phase as cofactors in neural injury induced by electrical stimulation. IEEE Trans Biomed Eng 1990;37:996–1001.

74   Huang CQ, Carter PM, Shepherd RK: Stimulus induced pH changes in cochlear implants: an in vitro and in vivo study. Ann Biomed Eng 2001;29:791–802.

75   Rose TL, Robblee LS: Electrical stimulation with Pt electrodes. VIII. Electrochemically safe charge injection limits with 0.2 ms pulses. IEEE Trans Biomed Eng 1990;37:1118–1120.

76   Brummer SB, Turner MJ: Electrical stimulation with Pt electrodes: II-estimation of maximum surface redox (theoretical non-gassing) limits. IEEE Trans Biomed Eng 1977;24:440–443.

77   Robblee LS, Lefko J, Brummer SB: Activated Ir: an electrode suitable for reversible charge injection in saline solution. J Electrochem Soc 1983;130:731–733.

78   Beebe X, Rose TL: Charge injection limits of activated iridium oxide electrodes with 0.2 m pulses in bicarbonate buffered saline. IEEE Trans Biomed Eng 1988;35:494–495.

79   McGinn MD, Faddis BT: Exposure to low frequency noise during rearing induces spongiform lesions in gerbil cochlear nucleus: high frequency exposure does not. Hear Res 1994;81:57–65.

80   McCreery DB, Agnew WF, Yuen TG, Bullara LA: Relationship between stimulus amplitude, stimulus frequency and neural damage during electrical stimulation of sciatic nerve of cat. Med Biol Eng Comput 1995;33(3 Spec No):426–429.

81   Colletti V, Carner M, Miorelli V, Guida M, Colletti L, Fiorino F: Auditory brainstem implant (ABI): new frontiers in adults and children. Otolaryngol Head Neck Surg 2005;133:126–138.

Robert K. Shepherd, PhD
Bionic Ear Institute
384–388 Albert Street
East Melbourne 3002, Victoria (Australia)
Tel. +61 3 99298397, Fax +61 3 96631958, E-Mail rshepherd@bionicear.org

Møller AR (ed): Cochlear and Brainstem Implants.
Adv Otorhinolaryngol. Basel, Karger, 2006, vol 64, pp 206–223

....

Physiological Basis for Cochlear and Auditory Brainstem Implants

Aage R. Møller

School of Behavioral and Brain Sciences, University of Texas at Dallas,
Richardson, Tex., USA

Abstract

Cochlear implants bypass functions of the cochlea that have been regarded to be fundamental for discrimination of the frequency (or spectrum). Frequency discrimination is essential for discrimination of sounds, including speech sounds, and the normal auditory system is
assumed to make use of both (power) spectral and temporal information for frequency discrimination. Spectral information is represented by the place on the basilar membrane that
generates the largest amplitude of vibration on the basilar membrane. Evidence has been presented that the temporal representation of frequency is more robust than the place representation and thus regarded more important for speech discrimination. The fact that some cochlear
implants provide good speech discrimination using only information about the energy in a few
spectral bands seems to contradict these studies. In that way, frequency discrimination may be
similar to trichromatic color vision, which is based on the energy in only three different
spectral bands of light, accomplished by different color-sensitive pigments in the cones of the
retina. Cochlear nucleus implants (ABIs) also bypass the auditory nerve, which does not perform any processing. Therefore, it may be expected that ABIs are equally efficient as cochlear
implants. However, experience from the use of ABIs in patients with bilateral vestibular
schwannoma has not been encouraging, but recent studies of the use of ABIs in patients with
other causes of injuries to the auditory nerve have shown similar speech discrimination as
achieved with modern cochlear implants. Cochlear implants and ABIs are successful in providing speech discrimination because of redundancy in the processing in the ear, redundancy
of the speech signal and because the auditory nervous system has a high degree of plasticity.
Expression of neural plasticity makes the auditory nervous system adapt to the change in
demands of processing of the information provided by cochlear implants.

Cochlear implants bypass the normal function of the cochlea, and the processors in these devices are designed to replace functions of the cochlea that are
regarded important for discrimination of sounds, foremost speech sounds. Modern

cochlear implants provide useful hearing without replacing the function of the cochlea completely and without providing the same coding of sounds in the auditory nerve as that of the normal cochlea. The emphasis has been on providing information about both the temporal and spectral aspects of sounds, and more recently cochlear implant processors that only provide spectral information have become in common use [Loizou, this vol, pp 109–143]. Cochlear implants are mainly aimed at establishing adequate speech discrimination, and only recently has attention been directed to other kinds of sounds, such as music sounds.

When Dr. House first introduced the cochlear implant using a single electrode it was met with great skepticism because it seemed unlikely that such a simple device could in any way replace the intricate and complex function of the cochlea. Even the function of modern multichannel cochlear implants that provide some spectral and temporal information seems crude compared to that of the normal cochlea, and indeed, they replace only some functions of the cochlea, and incompletely.

There are three main reasons why cochlear implants are successful in providing speech intelligibility and identification of environmental sound despite the fact that they do not replace all the functions of the normal cochlea: (1) Much of the natural speech signals are redundant. (2) Much of the normal processing capabilities of the ear are redundant. (3) Much of the processing that normally occurs in the auditory nervous system is redundant. (4) The central nervous system has an enormous ability to adapt ('re-wire') to changing demands through expression of neural plasticity.

The fact that much of the speech signal is redundant explains why cochlear implants only need to transmit a small fraction of the information that is contained in speech sounds to achieve good speech intelligibility. This was recognized as early as 1928 when Dudley conceived the 'vocoder' for transmitting speech over telephone lines [1] and this observation has been confirmed in many later studies [Loizou, this vol, pp 109–143].

Vocoders (the name derived from VOice and CODER) were developed because bandwidth was expensive at the time when copper wires were used in long telephone cables such as transoceanic cables. Now, these principles have found use in cochlear and cochlear nucleus implants. Other schemes emerged for compression of speech with regard to the bandwidth [2] but none of these systems were ever realized because of the availability of satellites and later fiber optic cables which offered inexpensive and reliable bandwidth that became available before vocoder systems could be realized into practical telephone systems. Before cochlear implants became in use, vocoders were used for developing devices for speech communication using the tactile sense [3].

It was earlier assumed that the complex function of the cochlea as a spectrum analyzer was the basis for the place hypothesis for frequency discrimination and that the neural coding of the temporal pattern of sounds was the basis for the temporal hypothesis of frequency discrimination. Both of these kinds of coding provided by the cochlea were assumed to be essential for discrimination of sounds such as speech sounds. The redundancy of these different kinds of analysis and coding of sounds in the ear were not fully appreciated before the results of studies of cochlear implants were available, although speech research had shown many years earlier that good speech discrimination could be achieved from spectral information only [1], thus based on the place hypothesis of frequency discrimination only. However, the experience from cochlear implants has confirmed these early results and brought new aspects on the functional importance of the analysis that occurs in the normal ear and the coding of sounds that occur in the auditory nerve. That the nervous system is plastic can explain why cochlear implants can provide adequate speech discrimination even though the coding of speech by cochlear implant processors is less sophisticated than that of the normal ear and why the use of different principles of coding can result in similar degree of speech discrimination.

The auditory nervous system is far more important for discrimination of sounds than generally recognized, and its capabilities to reorganize and the extent of redundancy in neural processing in the ascending auditory pathways, including the cerebral cortex, were likewise underestimated before experience of the performance of cochlear implants.

One aspect of the redundancy of the processing in the normal ear and auditory nervous system was demonstrated in psychoacoustic studies [1, 4, 5]. These studies showed that speech discrimination could be achieved on the basis of only spectral information or on the basis of only temporal information. That can explain why different processing schemes for cochlear implant processors can achieve similar speech discrimination abilities.

In this paper we will discuss the physiological basis for cochlear and cochlear nucleus implants. We will focus on frequency discrimination and discuss why cochlear and cochlear nucleus processors that are based on different principles can provide good speech discrimination. The similarity between auditory frequency discrimination using only power spectral cues and color vision will be discussed. Hypotheses about the differences in performance of auditory brainstem implants (ABIs) in NF2 patients and in patients with other causes of auditory nerve dysfunction are also discussed.

Auditory Frequency Discrimination: Place or Temporal Hypotheses?

Providing frequency discrimination is a prominent feature of the ear and the auditory nervous system and it is assumed to be important for speech discrimination, although changes in amplitude and duration of sounds and gaps between sounds are also important for discrimination of speech sounds. Much attention has therefore been devoted to find the anatomical and physiological bases for auditory frequency discrimination.

The ear provides two different codes of the frequency of sounds to the auditory nervous system, namely information about the (power) spectrum of sounds and about the waveform of sounds (temporal pattern) [for details about the anatomy and physiology of the cochlea, see 6]. Physically, the frequency (or spectrum) of sounds can be determined equally well from the result of spectral analysis such as that performed by the cochlea, as from analysis of the time pattern of sounds. This means that information about the frequency (or spectrum) of sounds can be derived from both of these two types of coding of sounds, which are the basis for the place hypothesis and the temporal hypothesis for frequency discrimination, respectively. Frequency analysis in the cochlea is the basis for the place hypothesis, and coding of the temporal pattern of sounds in the discharge pattern of auditory nerve fibers is the basis for the temporal hypothesis [6].

There is ample evidence from animal experiments that frequency is normally coded in the discharge pattern of single auditory nerve fibers, both as a temporal and a place code. Frequency tuning is a characteristic feature of nerve cells throughout the ascending classical auditory nervous system, and nerve cells in the ascending auditory pathways are organized anatomically according to the frequency to which they are tuned (tonotopical organization). There is less evidence, however, regarding which of these two ways of coding frequency is used as a basis for frequency discrimination in the normal auditory system. Still, psychoacoustic studies show that good speech discrimination can be achieved by either one of these two types of frequency coding [4, 5].

While the tonotopic organization in animals with normal hearing has been regarded to be the result of the tuning of the basilar membrane, recent studies showed that a rudimentary tonotopic organization exists in the nervous system in animals that are born deaf [7, 8]. Other studies have shown that organization can be refined through expression of neural plasticity elicited by sound stimulation [8, 9] and electrical stimulation of the cochlea can modify the cochleotropic organization that exists even in animals that never have had any auditory input [10–12]. It is assumed that the rudimentary tonotopic organization that exists at birth is normally refined by the sound that a child experiences through expression of neural plasticity.

Animal experiments have shown that tonotopic maps of the auditory cortex change after sound stimulation [13] as well as other properties of such neurons [14]. Neurons may be 'tagged' by the properties (frequency, etc.) of the sounds that activate the neurons. Expression of neural plasticity makes it possible for cochlear and cochlear nucleus implants to impose a new tonotopic organization of the auditory nervous system. The ability of the nervous system to change its function is greatest in a short period after birth [15], which explains why it is easier for young individuals to adapt to cochlear implants than adults [10, 15, 16].

Proper training can improve the success of cochlear implants in adults. Recording of auditory evoked potentials (event-related potentials) [16] in individuals with cochlear implants has demonstrated that input from cochlear implants can change the function of the auditory nervous system.

Expression of neural plasticity is therefore important both for the normal organization of the auditory nervous system and for the ability of the nervous system to change its function such as is necessary for achieving the best possible function of cochlear and brainstem implants.

Relative Importance of Place and Temporal Coding of Speech Sounds

The place principle was earlier regarded by many investigators to be the basis of frequency discrimination, but more recent research has favored the temporal hypothesis for speech discrimination. It has been concluded that the place coding is not sufficiently robust to be the basis of normal frequency discrimination because it depends on the stimulus intensity [17–19]. Animal studies have indicated that place representation of formant frequencies is not sufficiently acute within physiologic sound levels (above 50 dB SPL) [20] but the temporal code is more robust than the place code for neural representation of vowels in the auditory nerve [21], thus supporting the temporal hypothesis for frequency discrimination.

Psychoacoustic studies have shown, however, that adequate frequency discrimination can be achieved on the basis of either the place principle or the temporal principle, and that individuals with normal hearing can understand speech solely on the basis of temporal information [4], as well as solely on the basis of spectral (place) information [1, 2]. That frequency discrimination can be achieved on the basis of either the place or the temporal hypothesis is an example of the extensive redundancy of the auditory system.

Another hypothesis regarding the role of spectral filtering in the cochlea suggests that the division of the spectrum facilitates temporal coding in the auditory nerve and its subsequent decoding in the ascending auditory pathways. That hypothesis assumes that the most important function of the normal cochlea is to divide the spectrum of sound into 'slices' of suitable size, each of which

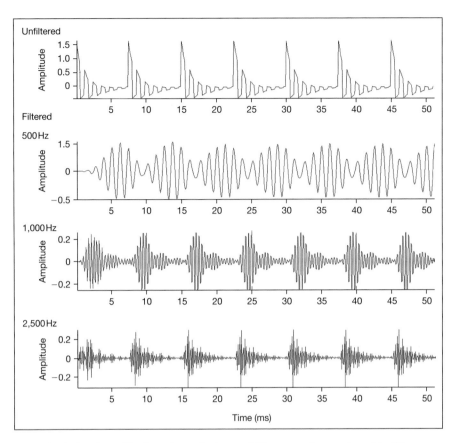

Fig. 1. Bandpass filtering of a synthetic vowel. The center frequencies of the filters were equal to the formant frequencies (500, 1,500, and 2,500 Hz). Courtesy of Peter Assmann and Ginger Stickly.

activates a specific population of cochlear hair cells which in turn excite specific populations of auditory nerve fibers. The waveform of such bandpass-filtered sounds that control the neural code in a population of auditory nerve fibers is much less complex than that of speech sounds that reach the ear (fig. 1).

This division of the sound spectrum is assumed to facilitate the temporal coding in single auditory nerve fibers, which become phase locked to a much less complex waveform than that of the sound wave that reaches the ear. It also reduces the demand on the encoding of the waveform of complex sounds, such as speech sounds. This is known as 'synchrony capture'.

Frequency Discrimination through Cochlear and Cochlear Nucleus Implants

All processors in cochlear implants and ABIs have a bank of bandpass filters that cover the frequency range that is most important for speech discrimination. Some cochlear implant processors extract a combination of spectral and temporal features for stimulation of auditory nerve fibers in the cochlea (compressed analog type processors [22] and continuous interleaved sampling [23]), while other types of cochlear implants use only spectral features together with low-frequency envelope information (vocoder type) [Loizou, this vol, pp 109–143 and 24, 25].

The implant devices that only provide information about the energy in 6–8 frequency bands resemble those of channel vocoders that were developed for analysis-synthesis telephony systems created in the 1950s and 1960s for the purpose of achieving economic speech transmission over long lines [2; see also Loizou, this vol, pp 109–143]. Cochlear implants that provide the temporal pattern within each frequency band in addition to spectral information (place information) stimulate auditory nerve fibers in a way that is more similar to that which the normal ear provides. However, cochlear implants using the vocoder principle seem equally efficient in providing good speech discrimination as those that also provide temporal information [26].

Channel Vocoder Type Processors

The vocoder type processors have a similar bank of bandpass filters as the CA type of processors, but the auditory nerve fibers are stimulated by electrical impulses that are controlled by the rectified and low-pass filtered output of the bandpass filters [Loizou, this vol, pp 109–143]. This means that most of the temporal information is thrown away and essentially only (power) spectral information of vowels is provided together with some low-frequency temporal information about the envelope of the output of each filter.

The success of cochlear implants that function as channel vocoders and do not use the temporal pattern of sounds seems to contradict the hypothesis that temporal information is important for speech discrimination. The question is therefore: how can only information about the energy in a few broad frequency bands provide enough information to establish good speech discrimination?

Analogy between Channel Vocoder Type Cochlear Implants and Color Vision

Cochlear implants of the channel vocoder type have similarities with trichromatic color vision in humans. Trichromatic color discrimination is based

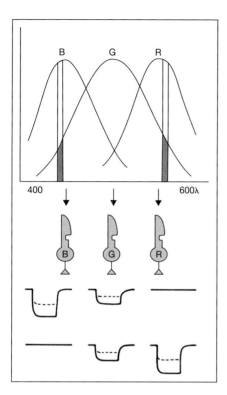

Fig. 2. Illustration of how a three-pigment system can distinguish colors (wavelength of light) independently of the intensity of the light, provided that the intensity is sufficient to elicit a response from at least two of the three kinds of receptors. Adapted from Shepherd [54].

on information about the light intensity in only three broad bands of the visual spectrum. Three kinds of photo pigment in the cones of the retina in the human eye act as spectral filters [27]. Trichromatic color vision using only the energy in three spectral bands provides the basis for discrimination of small nuances of color based on the fact that nuances of colors generate a unique combination of output in these three filters. This is similar to the channel vocoder type of cochlear implants that provide fine spectral discrimination of sounds that contain energy over a large frequency range based on the relationship between the output of a few spectral filters.

In the eye, the overall intensity of the light affects the activation of these three types of photo pigment equally and therefore does not affect the relationship between the output of the three receptors, and only the color (wavelength of light) will affect the relationship between the activation of the three types of photo pigments. The activation of the nerve fibers that innervate these three types of cones will thus be uniquely related to the spectrum of the light that reaches the eye (fig. 2).

This means that the relationship between the energy in these three bands of the visual spectrum provides sufficient information for discrimination between many nuances of colors and it is not necessary to have receptors that are sensitive to each wavelength of light that can be discriminated.

To illustrate how frequency discrimination in the auditory system can be achieved by using a few (3) filters, assume that the task is to determine the frequency of a pure tone, thus a single spectral component. When the bands of frequencies covered by each filter overlap as those of the eye (fig. 2), a tone with a frequency within the range covered by the filter bank, will cause output of more than one filter and the relationship between the output of the different filters will be unique for any frequency of the tone. It seems to be important that the different filters overlap so that a tone produces an output in more than one filter. It is probably also important that the filters have a rounded pass band rather than a flat top as is often preferred in man-made spectral filters.

The relationship between the outputs of a few filters can also provide information about the spectrum of broad sounds such as that of speech sounds; in the same way as the three spectral filters in the eye can provide information about the nuances of the color of light.

One of the strongest arguments against the place hypothesis for frequency discrimination has been its lack of robustness, consisting of a shift of the center frequency of cochlear filters and a widening of the filters that occur with increasing sound intensity [28, 29]. Since the bandpass filters in cochlear implant processors do not change with sound intensity, the vocoder-type cochlear implants may actually have an advantage over the cochlea as a frequency analyzer.

The Importance of Redundancy

The success of cochlear and cochlear nucleus implants depends on the redundancy in the processing in the cochlea and in the nervous system, and in natural sounds such as speech sounds. Only a small part of the speech wave is necessary for obtaining good intelligibility and this is why only spectral or only temporal information suffice to achieve good speech discrimination [2, 4].

Transmitting speech directly requires a bandwidth of approximately 3,000 Hz, but Dudley's channel vocoder could convert information about speech in a series control signal from which the speech could again be synthesized [Loizou, this vol, pp 109–143]. The bandwidth required for transmitting these signals was a small fraction of that required to transmit the speech signal, thus a sign of redundancy in the normal speech signal.

How Many Channels Are Necessary?

Development of the channel vocoder revealed that speech recognition does not require that fine spectral details are preserved [1, 2] and a total of 15 frequency bands was found to be sufficient for obtaining satisfactory speech intelligibly for telephone communication. The frequency analysis in the normal cochlea has been estimated to correspond to 28 independent filters [30], thus more than used in Dudley's channel vocoder and many more than the three filters that are the basis for trichromatic color vision. Speech intelligibility of cochlear implants that use the vocoder principle increases only slightly when the number of filters is increased above eight [31]. Studies in individuals with normal hearing where the vocoder principle has been simulated have shown that 4–5 channels are sufficient for a high degree of speech discrimination (90%), provided that a high degree of amplitude resolution is used [5, 32]. If the resolution of the coding of intensity is reduced, more channels are needed. Using 6 channels, the speech discrimination was reduced significantly when the intensity coding had only 8 steps and the number of channels had to be increased to 16 to obtain good speech discrimination (92%) with that resolution.

Coding of Sound Intensity

The function of cochlear implants that use the vocoder principle depends on proper coding of sound intensity in a wide range of sound intensities. Sound intensity is coded in auditory nerve fibers by the discharge rate, but only a few auditory nerve fibers seem to code sound intensity over the physiological range of sound intensities. The discharge rate of most nerve fibers reach saturation only 20–30 dB above hearing threshold [33]. Most nerve fibers, however, seem to code changes in sound intensity over a much larger range of sound intensities [34].

Cochlear implants code the intensity of sounds (the energy in respective frequency bands) by the amplitude of the electrical signals that are used to stimulate the auditory nerve. In the normal cochlea, increasing stimulus strength of a sound causes an increasing number of nerve fibers to become activated because of the widening of the segment of the basilar membrane that causes activation of nerve fibers [6]. In addition, the discharge rate at least of some nerve fibers increases with increasing stimulus intensity.

Functions Not Covered by Modern Cochlear Implants

Most modern cochlear implants generally do not convey information about the fine temporal pattern of sounds, and two-tone inhibition is not implemented in cochlear implants. The coding of the sounds in the discharge pattern of auditory nerve fibers is different from that provided by normal sound activation of hair cells; cochlear implants can activate many nerve fibers in a temporally coherent fashion.

Coding of the Temporal Pattern of Sounds

Modern cochlear implants of the vocoder type do not provide coding of the temporal pattern of sounds above 200 or 400 Hz [24, 25; see also Loizou, this vol, pp 109–143], thus fundamentally different from normal coding of sounds in the auditory nerve.

There are three different mechanisms for discrimination of pitch: place pitch, rate pitch and phase-locked pitch. Place pitch is based on the spectral filtering in the cochlea and rate pitch is based on coding of the temporal pattern of neural discharge in mostly a cycle-by-cycle manner and operates for low frequencies only. Phase-locked pitch is assumed to be based on temporal coding of the periodicity of sounds in a large range of frequencies. In the normal ear, all three forms of pitch perception may be utilized, but to a different degree for different sounds. It is evident that good speech discrimination can be achieved without preserving the temporal pattern of speech sounds such as vowels.

The performance of cochlear implants has mainly been judged on the basis of speech discrimination, but it has also been recognized that perception of music is inferior in cochlear implants [35–37]. While implant users perceive rhythm relatively well, melody recognition, perception of timbre and recognition of instruments are poor and implant users report that music is less pleasant than perceived by listeners with normal hearing [35]. The reason may be that music perception depends on coding of the fine temporal pattern of sounds such as what is assumed to be the basis for phase-locked pitch. The implant processors that use the continuous analog principle would be superior in that respect. New processing schemes that code periodicity have been shown to improve recognition of musical melody [38].

Two-Tone Suppression

In the normal auditory system, the response areas of auditory nerve fibers are surrounded by inhibitory bands [39], known as two-tone suppression [6]. Two-tone suppression that is a prominent property of the normal auditory system is not included in cochlear implants. It is believed that two-tone suppression may enhance spectral contrast in a similar way as lateral inhibition, which has been studied extensively in the visual system where it enhances contrast [40]. It is possible that two-tone inhibition in the auditory system enhances responses to sounds with rapidly varying frequency [41, 42].

Coherent Activation of Auditory Nerve Fibers

Cochlear implants cause temporal and spatially coherent activation of many nerve fibers, which is different from the normal activation of the auditory nerve. The importance of this is unknown but some hypotheses suggest that temporal coherence of activity in the auditory nerve is important for detection of sounds and for discrimination of sound intensity (loudness) [6].

Incorrect Stimulation of Nerve Fibers

Since the electrodes in cochlear implants are placed in the basal portion of the cochlea they do not stimulate auditory nerve fibers according to the frequencies to which they are normally tuned. The tonotopic maps on the nuclei of the ascending auditory pathways including the cerebral cortex will therefore be different in cochlear implant users than it is in individuals with normal hearing. Since the functional importance of the anatomical organization in individuals with normal hearing is unknown, it is also unknown what consequence different maps in cochlear implant users may have. Expression of neural plasticity is likely to correct these maps at least to some extent.

In the normal ear, the waves on the basilar membrane travel relatively slowly from the basal portion towards the apical portion of the basilar membrane and low-frequency components will normally activate nerve fibers later than high-frequency components. Cochlear implants do not take that difference in the travel times for low and high frequencies into account.

Cause of Variability in Performance of Cochlear Implants

The variability in performance of cochlear implants is considerable even within groups of individuals with similar age and with seemingly similar experience of previous sound exposure [26] (fig. 3). This variability is unexplained. The deviation in performance from the average performance may have different causes in different individuals; it may have to do with the amount of reserves that a person has, the size of which does not become apparent until the loss of hearing occurs. Differences in intellectual resources are likely to contribute to differences in performance of cochlear implants.

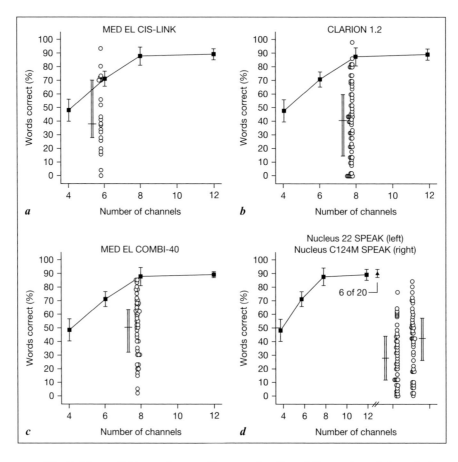

Fig. 3. Monosyllabic word recognition as a function of the number of channels in a signal processor for normal-hearing listeners (filled squares and solid lines). Performance of cochlear implant wearers is shown by open circles. The broad vertical lines indicate the interquartile range of performance. Horizontal bars indicate median scores. Reprinted from Møller [6] with permission from Elsevier. Data from Dorman [26].

Auditory Brainstem Implants

While ABIs in patients with NF2 provide assistance in lip-reading but no speech discrimination [43] recent experience shows that ABIs in patients with other causes of injuries to the auditory nerve can be equally efficient in providing speech comprehension as cochlear implants [44–47]. ABIs in children with malfunction of the auditory nerve such as may occur from internal auditory meatus malformation (atresia) causing auditory nerve aplasia also provide much better speech discrimination than those implanted in NF2 patients [Colletti, this vol, pp 167–185; 46].

Physiological Basis for ABIs

The main difference between cochlear implants and ABIs is that the latter also bypass the auditory nerve. The auditory nerve acts as a connection between the cochlea and the cochlear nucleus and does not perform any processing of information. Provided that proper placement of the stimulating electrode array on the surface of the cochlear nucleus can be arranged, ABIs can be expected to perform as well as cochlear implants. It is not known why ABIs do not provide useable speech discrimination in NF2 patients [43] but do much better in patients with other causes of auditory nerve malfunction [47]. Severance of the auditory nerve, often occurring in operations for large vestibular schwannoma, may affect the cells in the cochlear nucleus in a way that is different from what occurs in other forms of auditory nerve lesions. Animal experiments have shown that degeneration of nerve fibers that terminate on cells in the cochlear nucleus can result in changes in the cells in the cochlear nucleus [48, 49].

Anatomical Organization of the Cochlear Nucleus

The cochlear nucleus has three main divisions, the dorsal cochlear nucleus, the anterior ventral cochlear nucleus and the posterior ventral cochlear nucleus [6]. The surface of the ventral cochlear nucleus and that of the dorsal cochlear nucleus share the floor of the lateral recess of the fourth ventricle. The anterior ventral nucleus occupies the most rostral part of the cochlear nucleus [50, 51]. Each auditory nerve fiber bifurcates and one of the branches bifurcates again, and these three branches connect to cells in one of the three divisions of the cochlear nucleus. This means that cells in each of the three divisions receive input from the same auditory nerve fibers [6]. This is the beginning of parallel processing that is prominent in the ascending auditory pathways. Since ABIs activate only one of the three divisions of the cochlear nucleus, only one of the parallel pathways to higher nervous centers becomes activated. The implications of that are unknown.

The three divisions of the cochlear nucleus have different anatomical organization and the responses of cells are different. The cells in the cochlear nucleus are interconnected in complex networks and the cells have excitatory and inhibitory influence on each other. It may be preferable to place the stimulating electrodes on the surface of the ventral cochlear nucleus because the cells of that division receive only few auditory nerve fibers (primary-like nerve cells) and, therefore, electrical stimulation of these cells would be similar to stimulating auditory nerve fibers. However, electrical stimulation of the cochlear nucleus can stimulate different types of cells. Electrical stimulation from ABIs is less likely to activate nerve fibers within the cochlear nucleus [Shepherd and McCreery, this vol, pp 186–205].

The cochlear nucleus is tonotopically organized [6, 52], but it is not known if it is important to stimulate the cochlear nucleus cells according to this tonotopic organization. Since the orientation of the tonotopic maps of the cochlear nucleus in humans is insufficiently known, it is not possible to orient the electrode array so that frequency bands of the sound stimulate cells that are normally activated by the same spectrum of sounds.

While cochlear implants cannot stimulate auditory nerve fibers that normally respond to low-frequency sounds, ABIs can stimulate all neurons that normally respond to sounds within the entire audible hearing range, provided that the implanted electrode array is correctly placed. ABIs thereby have the potential of providing better hearing than cochlear implants.

Cause of Difference in Performance of ABIs in Patients with Different Cause of Auditory Nerve Injuries

The systematic difference in the performance of ABIs in NF2 patients and in patients with auditory nerve pathologies of other causes may have a specific cause, though yet unknown. Also, the performance of ABIs in NF2 patients varies and that may have causes similar to those discussed for cochlear implants (fig. 3).

The Role of Neural Plasticity

Since cochlear and cochlear nucleus implants do not accurately replace all the normal functions of the ear, the success of cochlear and cochlear nucleus implants implies that the nervous system must 'learn' a new code. Therefore, the success of cochlear implants and ABIs relies on functional adaptation of the processing of information in the auditory nervous system. Expression of neural plasticity enables the auditory nervous system to adapt to changing demands and it has been known for a long time that expression of neural plasticity helps to regain function after trauma or insults, such as from strokes [53]. Training is a powerful method for activating neural plasticity and a part of all cochlear and cochlear nucleus implant programs. These matters are discussed in papers by Sharma and Dorman [this vol, pp 66–88] and Kral and Tillein [this vol, pp 89–108].

References

1   Dudley H: Remaking speech. J Acoust Soc Am 1939;11:169–177.
2   Schroeder M: Vocoders: analysis and synthesis of speech. Proc IEEE 1966;54:720–734.
3   Pickett JM: Advances in sensory aids for the hearing-impaired: visual and vibrotactile aids. Ann Otol Rhinol Laryngol 1980;89:74–78.
4   Shannon RV, Zeng F-G, Kamath V, Wygonski J, Ekelid M: Speech recognition with primarily temporal cues. Science 1995;270:303–304.
5   Dorman M, Loizou P, Rainey R: Speech intelligibility as a function of the number of channels of stimulation for signal processors using sine-wave and noise-band outputs. J Acoust Soc Am 1997;102:2403–2411.
6   Møller AR: Hearing: Anatomy, Physiology and Disorders of the Auditory System, ed 2. Amsterdam, Elsevier, 2006.
7   Hartmann R, Shepherd RK, Heid S, Klinke R: Response of the primary auditory cortex to electrical stimulation of the auditory nerve in the congenitally deaf white cat. Hear Res 1997;112: 115–133.
8   Leake PA, Snyder RL, Rebscher SJ, Moore CM, Vollmer M: Plasticity in central representation in the inferior colliculus induced by chronic single- vs. two-channel electrical stimulation by cochlear implant after neonatal deafness. Hear Res 2000;147:221–241.
9   Snyder RL, Rebscher SJ, Cao K, Leake PA: Effects of chronic intracochlear stimulation in the neonatally deafened cat: I. Expansion of central spatial representation. Hear Res 1990;50:7–33.
10 Kral A, Hartmann R, Tillein J, Heid S, Klinke R: Hearing after congenital deafness: central auditory plasticity and sensory deprivation. Cereb Cortex 2002;12:797–807.
11 Klinke R, Hartmann R, Heid S, Tillein J, Kral A: Plastic changes in the auditory cortex of congenitally deaf cats following cochlear implantation. Audiol Neurootol 2001;6:203–206.
12 Kral A, Tillein J, Heid S, Hartmann R, Klinke R: Postnatal cortical development in congenital auditory deprivation. Cereb Cortex 2005;15:552–562.
13 Kilgard MP, Merzenich MM: Cortical map reorganization enabled by nucleus basalis activity. Science 1998;279:1714–1718.
14 Kilgard MP, Merzenich MM: Plasticity of temporal information processing in the primary auditory cortex. Nature Neurosci 1998;1:727–731.
15 Kral A, Hartmann R, Tillein J, Heid S, Klinke R: Delayed maturation and sensitive periods in the auditory cortex. Audiol Neurootol 2001;6:346–362.
16 Sharma A, Dorman MF, Kral A: The influence of a sensitive period on central auditory development in children with unilateral and bilateral cochlear implants. Hear Res 2005;203: 134–143.
17 Honrubia V, Ward PH: Longitudinal distribution of the cochlear microphonics inside the cochlear duct (guinea pig). J Acoust Soc Am 1968;44:951–958.
18 Møller AR: Review of the roles of temporal and place coding of frequency in speech discrimination. Acta Otolaryngol 1999;119:424–430.
19 Zwislocki JJ: What is the cochlear place code for pitch? Acta Otolaryngol 1992;111: 256–262.
20 Sachs MB, Young ED: Encoding of steady-state vowels in the auditory nerve: representation in terms of discharge rate. J Acoust Soc Am 1979;66:470–479.
21 Young ED, Sachs MB: Representation of steady-state vowels in the temporal aspects of the discharge patterns of populations of auditory nerve fibers. J Acoust Soc Am 1979;66:1381–1403.
22 Eddington D: Speech discrimination in deaf subjects with cochlear implants. J Acoust Soc Am 1980;68:885–891.
23 White M, Merzenich M, Gardi J: Multichannel cochlear implants: channel interaction and processor design. Arch Otolaryngol 1984;110:493–501.
24 Loizou PC: Introduction to cochlear implants. IEEE Signal Process Mag 1998;5:101–130.

25 Loizou P, Stickney G, Mishra L, Assmann P: Comparison of speech processing strategies used in the Clarion implant processor. Ear Hear 2003;24:12–19.

26 Dorman MF: Speech Perception by Adults; in Walzman C (ed): Cochlear Implants. New York, Thieme, 2000.

27 Møller AR: Sensory Systems: Anatomy and Physiology. Amsterdam, Academic Press, 2003.

28 Møller AR: Frequency selectivity of single auditory nerve fibers in response to broadband noise stimuli. J Acoust Soc Am 1977;62:135–142.

29 Zwislocki JJ: What is the cochlear place code for pitch? Acta Otolaryngol 1991;111:256–262.

30 Moore BC: Coding of sounds in the auditory system and its relevance to signal processing and coding in cochlear implants. Otol Neurotol 2003;24:243–254.

31 Fishman KE, Shannon RV, Slattery WH: Speech recognition as a function of the number of electrodes used in the SPEAK cochlear implant speech processor. J Speech Lang Hear Res 1997;40: 1201–1215.

32 Loizou PC: On the number of channels needed to understand speech. J Acoust Soc Am 1999;106: 2097–2103.

33 Müller M, Robertson D, Yates GK: Rate-versus-level functions of primary auditory nerve fibres: evidence of square law behavior of all fibre categories in the guinea pig. Hear Res 1991;55:50–56.

34 Cooper NP, Robertson D, Yates GK: Cochlear nerve fiber responses to amplitude-modulated stimuli: variations with spontaneous rate and other response characteristics. J Neurophysiol 1993; 70:370–386.

35 McDermott HJ: Music perception with cochlear implants: a review. Trends Amplif 2004;8:49–82.

36 Gfeller K, Olszewski C, Rychener M, Sena K, Knutson JF, Witt S, Macpherson B: Recognition of 'real-world' musical excerpts by cochlear implant recipients and normal-hearing adults. Ear Hear 2005;26:237–250.

37 Loeb GE: Are cochlear implant patients suffering from perceptual dissonance? Ear Hear 2005;26: 435–450.

38 Laneau J, Wouters J, Moonen M: Improved music perception with explicit pitch coding in cochlear implants. Audiol Neurootol 2005;11:38–52.

39 Sachs MB, Kiang NYS: Two tone inhibition in auditory nerve fibers. J Acoust Soc Am 1968;43:1120–1128.

40 Ratliff F: Mach Bands. Quantitative Studies on Neural Networks in the Retina. San Francisco, Holden-Day, Inc., 1965.

41 Møller AR: Coding of sounds with rapidly varying spectrum in the cochlear nucleus. J Acoust Soc Am 1974;55:631–640.

42 Eggermont JJ: Between sound and perception: reviewing the search for a neural code. Hear Res 2001;157:1–42.

43 Lenarz M, Matthies C, Lesinski-Schiedat A, Frohne C, Rost U, Illg A, Battmer RD, Samii M, Lenarz T: Auditory brainstem implant part II: subjective assessment of functional outcome. Otol Neurotol 2002;23:694–697.

44 Colletti V, Carner M, Miorelli V, Colletti L, Guida MFF: Auditory brainstem implant in posttraumatic cochlear nerve avulsion. Audiol Neurootol 2004;9:247–255.

45 Colletti V, Fiorino FG, Sacchetto L, Miorelli V, Carner M: Hearing habilitation with auditory brainstem implantation in two children with cochlear nerve aplasia. Int J Pediatr Otorhinolaryngol 2001;60:99–111.

46 Colletti V, Carner M, Fiorino F, Sacchetto L, Morelli V, Orsi A, Cilurzo F, Pacini L: Hearing restoration with auditory brainstem implant in three children with cochlear nerve aplasia. Otol Neurotol 2002;23:682–693.

47 Colletti V, Shannon RV: Open set of speech perception with auditory brainstem implant? Laryngoscope 2005;115:1974–1978.

48 Sie KCY, Rubel EW: Rapid changes in protein synthesis and cell size in the cochlear nucleus following eighth nerve activity blockade and cochlea ablation. J Comp Neurol 1992;320: 501–508.

49 Deitch JS, Rubel EW: Rapid changes in ultrastructure during deafferentiation-induced dendritic atrophy. J Comp Neurol 1989;281:234–258.

50   Kuroki A, Møller AR: Microsurgical anatomy around the foramen of Luschka with reference to intraoperative recording of auditory evoked potentials from the cochlear nuclei. J Neurosurg 1995;933–939.

51   Terr LI, Edgerton BJ: Surface topography of the cochlear nuclei in humans: two and three-dimensional analysis. Hear Res 1985;17:51–59.

52   Rose JE, Galambos R, Hughes JR: Microelectrode studies of the cochlear nuclei in the cat. Bull Johns Hopkins Hosp 1959;104:211–251.

53   Møller AR: Neural plasticity and disorders of the nervous system. Cambridge, Cambridge University Press, 2006.

54   Shepherd GM: Neurobiology. New York, Oxford University Press, 1994.

Aage R. Møller, PhD
School of Behavioral and Brain Sciences
University of Texas at Dallas, GR 41
PO Box 830688
Richardson, TX 75083-0688 (USA)
Tel. +1 972 883 2313, Fax +1 972 883 2310, E-Mail amoller@utdallas.edu

Author Index

Subject Index